NEVER LET A GOOD DISASTER GO TO WASTE

NEVER LET A GOOD DISASTER GO TO WASTE

Making Sense of a Life of Absurdity
A Memoir

KAT FINNERTY

Never Let a Good Disaster Go To Waste: Making Sense of a Life of Absurdity

© Copyright 2023 Kat Finnerty

All rights reserved. No part of this publication may be reproduced, distributed or transmitted in any form or by any means, including photocopying, recording, or other electronic or mechanical methods, without the prior written permission of the publisher, except in the case of brief quotations embodied in critical reviews and certain other noncommercial uses permitted by copyright law.

Although the author and publisher have made every effort to ensure that the information in this book was correct at press time, the author and publisher do not assume and hereby disclaim any liability to any party for any loss, damage, or disruption caused by errors or omissions, whether such errors or omissions result from negligence, accident, or any other cause.

Adherence to all applicable laws and regulations, including international, federal, state and local governing professional licensing, business practices, advertising, and all other aspects of doing business in the US, Canada or any other jurisdiction is the sole responsibility of the reader and consumer.

Neither the author nor the publisher assumes any responsibility or liability whatsoever on behalf of the consumer or reader of this material. Any perceived slight of any individual or organisation is purely unintentional.

The resources in this book are provided for informational purposes only and should not be used to replace the specialised training and professional judgment of a health care or mental health care professional.

Neither the author nor the publisher can be held responsible for the use of the information provided within this book. Please always consult a trained professional before making any decision regarding treatment of yourself or others.

Contact Kat Finnerty - Email: katfinnerty@hotmail.com

Website: www.katfinnerty.com

ISBN: 979-8-88759-563-4 - paperback

ISBN: 979-8-88759-564-1 - ebook

ISBN: 979-8-88759-996-0 - hardcover

Contents

Chapter 1: Curiosity Killed the Kat........................1
Chapter 2: Overcoming Betrayal in 12 Hours............15
Chapter 3: 12 Principles for a Happier Life...............25
Chapter 4: The Child Who Should Have Been Drowned at Birth........................31
Chapter 5: Affection Is Reserved for the Italians..........37
Chapter 6: The Flipside of Pleasure Is Pain...............47
Chapter 7: Tiny but Tuff................................53
Chapter 8: Let Go and Let God.........................61
Chapter 9: Toughen Up Buttercup......................73
Chapter 10: The Cult of Personality......................81
Chapter 11: The Bachelor Auction.......................91
Chapter 12: Feel the Fear and Do It Anyway.............101
Chapter 13: Island of the Gods.........................107
Chapter 14: Life Is But a Dream........................119
Chapter 15: Fate, Destiny or Karma....................129
Chapter 16: Everything I Never Wanted................141
Chapter 17: No More Itch to Scratch...................149
Chapter 18: The Sleeping Dragon Awakes...............163
Chapter 19: Fake It 'Til You Make It....................175
Chapter 20: A Taste of the Past........................181
Chapter 21: Surviving the Shoah.......................191
Chapter 22: My First Best Mistake.....................205
Chapter 23: A Slippery Slope into a Black Hole.........213
Chapter 24: The Blissful Pursuit of Ignorance...........223
Chapter 25: The Miracle of Spandex...................229

Chapter 26:	A Cry For Help	239
Chapter 27:	Wisdom from a Warrior Princess	245
Chapter 28:	How Vegemite Changed My Life	255
Chapter 29:	Planting the Seeds of Good Karma	261
Chapter 30:	A Spiritual Renegade's Guide to the Good Life	269
Chapter 31:	It's Like This Now	277
Chapter 32:	The MS Roller Coaster	283
Chapter 33:	Salvation in the Promised Land	289
Chapter 34:	The Road to Recovery	301
Chapter 35:	Liberation Therapy	311
Chapter 36:	Life After Life	321
Chapter 37:	Releasing the Karma Genie	325
Chapter 38:	The Five Rs	329
Chapter 39:	Love Is a Verb as Well as a Noun	333
Chapter 40:	A Backpack Full of Bowling Balls	337
Chapter 41:	Struggling With My Big Girl Pants	343
Chapter 42:	Running Out of Kat Lives	349
Chapter 43:	The Domino Effect	357
Chapter 44:	Zombie Apocalypse	365
Chapter 45:	Bake a Cake for Someone You Hate	371
Chapter 46:	A Shamanic Brush with Elizabeth Gilbert	379
Chapter 47:	Serendipity and Chocolate Cake	385
Chapter 48:	It Starts with a Belief	393
Chapter 49:	Never Let a Good Disaster Go to Waste	399
Chapter 50:	Tales of the South Pacific	405

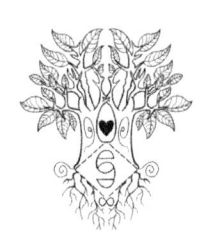

Foreword

Laurentine ten Bosch,
Co-founder of Food Matters (foodmatters.com)

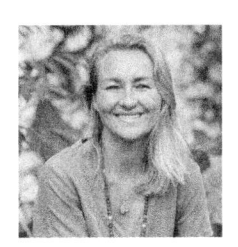

Oh my gosh…I'm totally speechless! This story moved me from laughing (because yes, this is Kat's authentic self) to crying and yelling out loud (from a maternal and protective aspect), to a cheerleader supporting her struggles being the warrior woman she truly is. As the snippets of Kat's life journey unfolded, I sat in total awe.

For those that are struggling with a chronic illness or looking to overcome challenge and adversity, this inspiring book will change your outlook on life and equip you with tools to help you navigate them. Kat tells her personal life story and weaves in an array of philosophies and daily practices that, if adopted, will transform your health and life. This memoir proves that there is always a way out of the proverbial "Rabbit Hole".

Lama Marut (1953 - 2019)
www.lamamarut.org

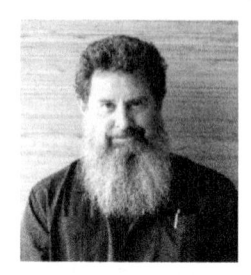

"In this life, we are either in a disaster or between them. And so a spiritual renegade is someone who has wised up a bit, who has dropped the delusion that they are somehow uniquely protected from suffering…and is willing to roll up his or her sleeves and do the hard work of making some inner changes so that they will be able to deal effectively with whatever life throws at them."

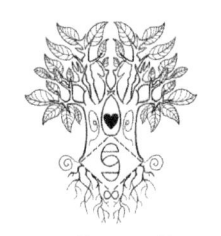

Dedication

To my father for not drowning me, to my mother for saving me, to my children for teaching me, to my siblings for their unconditional love, to my husband for betraying me, to Alex for his infinite patience, to my spiritual teachers for guiding me out of suffering—and finally to all of my 'Kat'astrophes, thank you, for showing me why I should never let a good disaster go to waste.

This memoir is my interpretation of the events that have occurred in my life. As such, I have taken the liberty of making some minor tweaks, changes and additions to enhance flow, timelines, dialogue and story-lines. Some names and places have been changed for privacy purposes.

Definition: **Absurd** - wildly unreasonable

'In conclusion, human life is naturally absurd, due to its being characterised by suffering, death and an absence of meaning. However, it may become otherwise as one may 'stamp' meaning onto life through compassion and striving for 'Superman' status. Doing so enables, and may provide, happiness.'

Is Human Life Absurd? Abstract by Billy Holmes.

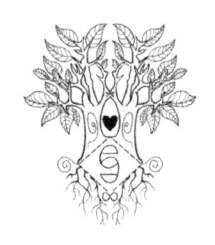

My Free Gift To You

Head to my website www.katfinnerty.com to download a free summary and breakdown of my **12 PRINCIPLES** of how to become a *Master of Disaster*. These powerful principles are the key to helping you overcome and transform any adversity or betrayal, no matter how painful, in as little as 12 hours!

As part of my Masters of Disaster (MOD) Community you'll receive amazing discounts, deals and insider access to my upcoming books, courses, blogs and retreats. There's also a free download available of the first chapter of my companion self-help book, *How to Get Over Betrayal in 12 Hours*: *A Survival Manual for the Soul*

The 12 Principles

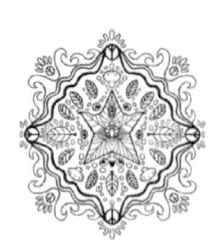

Use Gratitude As
A Game Changer

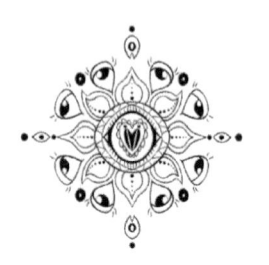

Become A
Maestro Of
Manifestation

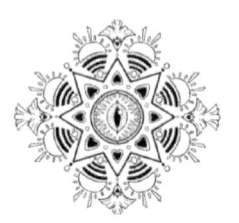

Find A Purpose
In The Pain

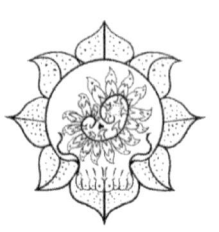

Acknowledge
Impermanence

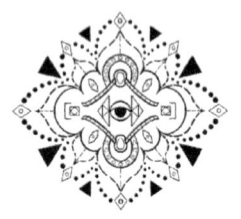

Unleash The
Power Of
Perception

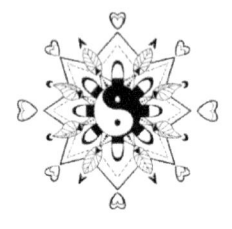

Enable Empathy
& Compassion

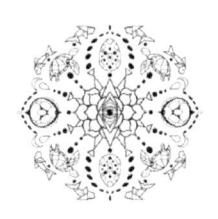

Embrace Radical Forgiveness

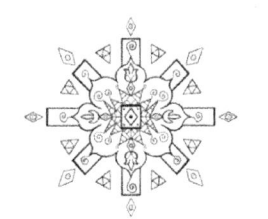

Cast Off The Mantle Of Victimhood

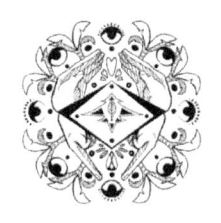

Respond With Radical Acceptance

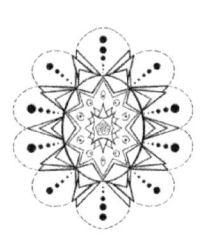

Take Action To Create Better Karma

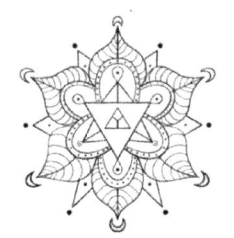

Master Your Thoughts

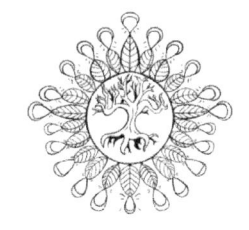

Let Go Of Unhealthy Attachments

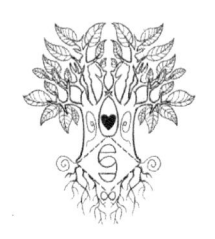

Never Let a Good Disaster Go To Waste

Making Sense of a Life of Absurdity
A Memoir

By Kat Finnerty

My story is cut with raw edges,
questionable choices
and destructive behaviours.
It also features a
radical transformation
and a shift in perception
that saved my life
and placed peace in my heart.
Never let a good disaster go to waste.

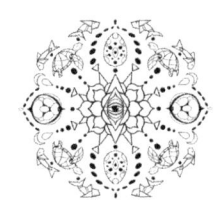

CHAPTER ONE
Curiosity Killed the Kat

*You can choose to suffer for 12 hours, 12 days,
12 years, or a lifetime. I chose 12 hours.
~ Kat Finnerty*

I'm sitting on my bedroom floor, numb and in shock. It's been ten hours since I was lying on an operating table in Melbourne's Alfred Hospital. Trevor's words are reverberating inside my head. 'It's over, I'm leaving you, I love her.'

Imagine for your 40th birthday, instead of breakfast in bed and cuddles from your children, you're about to be wheeled into an operating room, a human guinea pig for a controversial and risky medical experiment. The procedure involved inserting a thin catheter into my thigh and threading it carefully through my body up into my neck. There, a tiny balloon would be inflated to expand my jugular and increase blood flow from my brain to my body.

It was September 2012. Melbourne was just coming out of a harsh winter, Julia Gillard was making history as Australia's first female Prime Minister, and I had been battling a crippling illness for almost half my life. According to my doctors, I should have been confined to a wheelchair by now. But amazingly, I'd been in remission for around five years, thanks to my unrelenting efforts to find a cure for my incurable disease. I was still far from what most people would consider 'normal'. Countless attacks over the years had left their hidden, internal scars on me and the chance of a relapse and the threat of permanent disability perpetually hung over my head like a guillotine. Hence why I'd thrown my hat in the ring to be part of the research trial.

I felt my mobile vibrating on the bed next to me. It was my ten-year-old daughter, Stella.

'Morning Mummy,' she chimed in a sing-song voice.

My heart warmed. Stella proceeded to sing me 'Happy Birthday', then excitedly announced, 'And guess what Mummy?'

'Yes darling?'

'Tahlia slept over in your bed last night!'

'Oh...really?'

'Ya, Daddy slept on the couch.'

I hesitated as I tried to process this.

'Of course he did. Have a great day at school honey. Love you.'

My hand holding the phone trembled slightly as I forced out a cheerful goodbye.

I should have seen it coming. Major disasters always happen on my birthday. Death, incredible pain, disease—I've come to the realisation that it's all part of this game we call life. You know how curiosity killed the cat? Well, I was the 'Kat', and I was well on my way to using up every one of my nine lives. I'd spent decades dealing with my disasters and figuring out how to transform them into opportunities. Yet here I was, once again peering down the rabbit hole, wondering whether this was the start of a new 'Kat'astrophe or simply a colossal misunderstanding.

A nurse took me through the swinging doors into the brightly lit operating theatre. Sensing my unease, she leaned over and patted my hand.

'Don't you worry love. You'll be just fine.'

She had no idea the scalpel was the least of my worries. She continued to reassure me as she pushed me into the theatre, and then—oh my God, everything was not fine! There, smiling at me were two of the hottest male nurses I'd ever seen, their green scrubs nearly ripping over their bulging biceps. And here I was, embarrassingly attired in an unflattering blue hairnet and a hideous hospital gown. The two nurses helped me ever so gently from the gurney onto the table, while in the background Carly Rae Jepsen sang suggestively 'Call Me Maybe' through the overhead speakers.

'Hi, I'm Jared. You're in safe hands.'

'And I'm Brad. Let's get you comfortable.'

I thought I could quite possibly die happily right there and then. That's when I spotted the yellow plastic razor sitting on

3

the metal tray next to me. I was mortified. *Oh, sweet Jesus, one of these Adonis's is about to perform bush maintenance on my nether regions!* Nurse Jared followed my gaze and, with a sympathetic grin, assured, 'Don't you worry, darlin'. I'll wait until you're well out of it before using that.'

I turned and pleaded to the man sitting to my left. 'I think I need you.'

The anaesthetist chuckled as he depressed the syringe.

'Here comes the gin, and here comes the juice.'

I mercifully drifted off, relieved to be oblivious to whatever they were about to do to me.

When I finally came around, all I could think about was the phone conversation with my daughter. It played over and over again in my head. I needed to check out of the hospital ASAP and figure out what the hell was going on at home, and apparently, I needed to change my sheets. A woman wearing a familiar-looking blue hairnet pulled back the curtain and set down a tray of food in front of me. I removed the bread, made a sandwich of middles and drank lukewarm tea from a rose-coloured plastic mug. After getting dressed, I sat on the edge of my bed and gingerly picked at the tape holding the cannula in place. I buzzed for the nurse who appeared at my bedside looking perplexed, likely because I was dressed, my bed was made and my bag was packed.

She frowned. 'Everything okay here?'

'Yes, I'm feeling perfectly fine,' I explained apologetically, 'but my sister had to come early to pick me up. Her daughter was vomiting at school. They're downstairs waiting for me. I'm sorry, but I need to leave. Could you please take the needle out of my arm?'

I crossed my fingers behind my back, hoping she wouldn't guess I was fibbing.

'I'll ask the doctor, but you're meant to be here for another three hours.'

'I know, but honestly I feel fine and my sister's a nurse. She'll be with me the entire day.'

Oh dear, lie number two. But it sufficed to secure my early release.

As I began the four-hour drive through the traffic of Melbourne, heading north to the county, I was grateful for my uncanny ability to breeze through anaesthesia and recover rapidly. After all, I was no novice at this game. I tried listening to podcasts to pass the time but was far too distracted. A big knot had tied itself in my stomach and finally, it got the better of me. I worked up the courage to call Tahlia. She answered on the first ring.

'Happy birthday Kat! How'd it go?'

'I'm fine, other than my neck feeling like someone shoved a stick up inside of it.'

I hesitated before launching into my next question. 'Hey, uh, I spoke to Stella this morning and she told me you had a sleepover last night?'

'Oh…yeah. You wouldn't believe it,' she laughed. 'I popped in to say hi to Trev and the kids and we had a few too many wines. I got up to leave, then tripped over the ottoman and thought I'd better not drive.'

5

Really? You only live 800 metres away; you couldn't hit something if you tried. Do you really think it was a good idea to sleep at my house...in my bed?

At least that's what I wanted to say, but then it occurred to me that at some point in my life, I may have committed a similar drunken escapade. My memory had a habit of being advantageously selective.

Instead, I blurted out, 'Did you sleep well?'

Good grief, I sounded like a hotel concierge.

'Uh, yeah, okay I guess. But my head isn't great today. Hey, I still want to take you out for a birthday lunch. What day works for you?'

'Thanks Tal, but let's go for a walk tomorrow instead. Eating in the middle of the day involves devouring too many calories and too much sitting. I hope your head feels better soon,' I added, attempting to sound sincere.

'Thanks, enjoy the rest of your birthday. I'll see ya tomorrow.'

The knot began to unravel. Her explanation seemed plausible, and she sounded perfectly normal on the phone. Plus, she was a good friend who often dropped by. I concluded that being too drunk to drive was a perfectly valid excuse for a sleepover.

The city slowly began to melt away to be replaced by endless green paddocks, leaving me with plenty of time to mull over my marriage and my life. Trevor and I had been married for 14 years, and we were happy—well, except for all the times when we weren't—but we'd worked our way through most of our troubles. For an early 40th birthday present, Trevor surprised me by hiring a marquee for the annual local races and inviting our friends and his family along for the celebration.

Our hectic family life was also becoming easier thanks to the fact our three kids had nearly finished primary school. We were financially secure and looking forward to embarking on the next phase of our lives, which I fervently hoped would entail leaving Jrudgerie. Everything seemed to be sailing along smoothly. A few hours later, I received a text from my husband. It simply read 'Happy birthday old girl,' followed by one party popper emoji. No love hearts, no XXXs, no OOOs.

I made it home just before dusk and was greeted by one of those spectacular Aussie outback sunsets that seem to go on forever. It was a small consolation for living on the flat plains of Jrudgerie, where the view of the horizon stretched unobstructed for hundreds of kilometres. Soon I would be greeted with an equally spectacular moonrise.

As I walked into the house, I was greeted by Trevor dashing out the door with our daughter in tow.

'Hey, you're home early! We'll be right back. We haven't fed Belle yet.'

Belle was Stella's horse who was agisted on a property at the edge of town. I went to the kitchen. On the table were remnants of their dinner—and Trevor's phone. In his haste, he'd forgotten to take it. I couldn't believe my luck. I grabbed the phone, along with a half-eaten chicken drumstick, and made my way to our bedroom. I started scrolling through his messages, absentmindedly chewing on what was left of the meat, thinking I had nothing to worry about.

That is, until I saw the messages between my husband and Tahlia. Time lurched to a halt. I gasped, nearly choking on the chicken. Their exchange was so explicit I wondered if they were submitting a short story to an adult magazine. The texts left very little to the imagination. There were also messages about how they would soon be living together on a beach with screenshots of glowing ocean sunsets. My heart began pounding as a nauseating, raw panic overwhelmed me.

'Oh my God!' I screamed. 'They're planning to escape Jrudgerie and leave me here!'

It seemed the person I'd vowed to be true to in good times and bad, for better or for worse, the person I would have taken a bullet for was now the one standing behind the gun pulling the trigger.

It soon became clear that some of our friends and even Trev's family were aware of the affair. One message mentioned how delighted his father was to see them so happy together. My broken heart shattered all over again. I had never felt so betrayed. I adored his parents and had even invited them on our honeymoon. Being deceived by my husband was devastating, but being betrayed by a family I cherished and loved like my own was soul-destroying. Trust, years to build seconds to break. How true.

I slid from the corner of the bed to the floor with a thud. It felt as if someone had punched me in the stomach, I couldn't breathe. My heart raced and my thoughts imploded. Fear, grief, pain, and rage tore through me and shredded me to my core. I didn't know whether to scream or curl into a ball and disappear forever. I violently threw the drumstick against the wall. It bounced onto the carpet, leaving behind a large, greasy stain. *Great! Another mess to clean up.* I opened the neck of my shirt and tried to slow my breathing as sweat dripped down my back. The whole scenario felt like a nightmare, except it was all too real. My mind was desperately grasping at straws as I tried to make sense of what I'd just discovered. There *had* to be a way of saving my marriage, my family…my life!

It was then I heard his car pull up. Unable to move, paralysed by fear. I sat on the carpet. Waiting.

The front door opened and Stella yelled, 'Hey Mum, we're back.' Trevor's heavy footsteps echoed down the hall. I wondered if he realised he'd left his phone behind yet. When he passed the open door to our bedroom, he glanced in and paused, taking in the scene. I lay slumped against the bed like a ragdoll, clutching his phone to my heart. I looked up, our eyes connected and in that moment he knew that I knew. In silence, he walked towards me, crouched down and prised his phone from my hands.

'It's over. I'm leaving you. I love her,' he stated with steely finality.

I didn't know what I was expecting, but it definitely wasn't this. Perhaps an apology, maybe a few excuses, a sorrowful admittance of his betrayal. Instead, I was served a brutal, final statement of his love for another woman and the resounding slam of the front door as he left. So, *this* was how it ended? A clichéd scene from an episode of *The Jerry Springer Show*? After 14 years of marriage and three children?

The irony of the situation rocked me. We lived in a town so boring I'd jokingly called it 'Jrudgerie', never by its true name, which was marginally less interesting. Nothing exciting had happened here since the Kelly gang arrived 140 years ago and robbed the bank. Scandals like this didn't happen to me, to my family, to this town. But now, of course, it had. Most hurtful was my mother-in-law's involvement in the whole sordid affair. She'd been like a mother to me. I loved her and thought the feeling was mutual. She often referred to me as her fourth daughter. As bad as it was having my husband admit he loved another woman, it didn't even begin to compare to the pain of her deception. This was apocalyptic.

My belly churned as I dialled her number. She answered cheerfully, 'Hi love, how are you?'

'Rosie, I…I know.' Emotions overwhelmed me as I choked to a halt.

'Oh honey, I'm so sorry, I wanted to speak to you, to tell you, but I just couldn't. Are you okay?'

'No,' I said shakily, 'I'm not okay.'

My world had just fallen apart, and the woman who I'd adored for 15 years had just admitted she'd known about the affair. Silence. A long pause. I could hear my mother-in-law attempting to hold back a sob.

'Kat, you know I love you. Everything will be okay. I'll come and see you first thing tomorrow.'

I breathed a small sigh of relief and said goodbye. For now, it seemed there was one less knife buried in my back.

I crawled over and picked up the chicken bone, rose to my feet and staggered down the corridor to my favourite room in the house, the kitchen. For once, I was grateful for the handheld technology that kept my daughter happily ensconced in her room. Tonight I had a much bigger problem to deal with than a Snapchat addiction. My nails dug into the counter as I looked up and silently screamed, 'What now?' When the Universe didn't reply, I did the only thing I could do in an emergency situation. I gathered together the Holy Trinity: chocolate, chips and wine. What ensued next was a battle of wills; a fierce stare down with the unopened bottle of merlot, a bar of Lindt and a bag of Ruffles. I swept them aside. Self-sabotage would not be the answer to this disaster.

Kat, you've studied Buddhism, meditation and yoga for over a decade. You've dealt with death, disability and disease. You've attended countless courses and studied innumerable texts about finding happiness. You've got this!

And somehow, as I uttered the words, I started to feel as if, maybe, just maybe, I did.

Throughout my life I've endured dozens of disasters. Each time, I've endeavoured to rationalise the situation by telling myself that this hasn't happened to me, it's happened for me, and that these were the lessons I needed to learn. However, this last disaster seemed truly 'Kat'astrophic'. Transcending it was going to be a huge task, even with my unique life history. I returned to my bedroom and gave myself a stern talking-to.

Come on girl, you can do this, even without booze. A journey of a thousand miles begins with one step, so take the damn step! I stepped.

I started by thinking about my cat. Yes, I know, a strange place to begin looking for enlightenment. But in addition to being curious, intelligent and independent, cats have an innate 'righting reflex', an ability to twist around in mid-air while falling and land on all fours. It's partly why they are gifted with the myth of nine lives. I figured what I really needed to do was to be more cat-like, or maybe Kat-like, by somehow finding a way to flip this situation into something good using my own 'righting reflex'.

As the darkest hours of the night ticked by, that's exactly what I did. I began comparing and analysing my current situation to all my past disasters, using the wisdom I'd collected over my 40 years to put things into perspective. It wasn't easy. Heavy waves of sadness kept crashing over me, dragging me down into a whirlpool of fear, anger, loss and grief and each time I struggled back up to the surface, my mind would gasp for a breath of calming air. With a supreme effort of willpower, I forced myself to mentally tread water and refocus on the bigger picture, ignoring the turbulence around me. *All that pain you've endured, everything you've overcome, don't let it go to waste Kat, don't let any of your disasters go to waste, especially this* one. There's a lesson hidden within this adversity; your mission is to find it.

And just like the jigsaw puzzles I used to do as a kid, the pieces started slotting into place. It was an empowering experience. I felt like Jamal in *Slumdog Millionaire*, only instead of winning a game show and a bucket load of cash, the Universe was miraculously conspiring to help me find the answers I was searching for and win at the game of life.

Sometime much later I noticed the sky starting to brighten outside, confirmation that I'd made it through the darkness and into the light. Gazing at the empty space where Trevor usually slept, I found I was wistful but not heart achingly sad. Hope had sprouted in my heart, and its powerful tendrils were slowly pushing out the anger and agony that had resided there just 12 hours earlier. I was no longer a devastated mess, thanks to the fact I'd asked myself over and over again, 'How long are you going to choose to suffer?'

A new day was beginning, a new door was opening and I wondered what the next chapter of my life held in store. As if on cue, a shaft of sunlight peeked over the horizon and illuminated my bedroom in a brilliant golden glow. I smiled.

The Universe had finally answered me.

CHAPTER TWO
Overcoming Betrayal in 12 Hours

Every new beginning comes from some other beginning's end.
~ Semisonic, Closing Time

Twelve hours, the average number of hours of light versus darkness on planet Earth. Twelve hours, the time elapsed since my husband threw me under a bus and replaced me with our friend Tahlia. Twelve hours, the length of suffering I endured after deciding that rather than drink the world dry of wine, I'd keep my head clear and contemplate the reality of the end of my marriage.

At some point in the night I realised I had a choice: I could suffer for 12 hours, 12 months, 12 years, or a lifetime. Having been to hell and back more times than I cared to count, I knew the length of my suffering was entirely up to me. So I chose 12 hours. I didn't have to view my husband's betrayal as a disaster. Rather, I could treat it as an opportunity to pursue a different life. My marriage may have ended and my old life was over, but now a new beginning awaited.

It was just past sunrise and my first client would be arriving shortly for his personal training session. As I made the bed, it hit me: I'd forgotten to change the sheets. I laughed as I tore them off the bed and threw them into the fire. Okay, so substitute hot wash for fire—no need to be irrational, they were my good sheets. I quickly showered, changed into my activewear and opened the door of the garage housing my yoga and fitness studio. My first client for the day was Bob, a wise old friend and an engineer used to solving complex problems. His wife had literally jumped the fence ten years before, shacking up with the neighbour, so I was hoping he'd have some sage advice for me.

When he walked in and asked how I was, I gave it to him straight.

'Trevor left me last night. He's in love with someone else.'

'What! No! Seriously?' He studied my face to see if I was joking. When he realised I wasn't he said, 'I'm so sorry Kat. Are you okay?'

I had to think about it for a few seconds before replying.

'To be perfectly honest, I was pretty devastated at first. I was angry and scared and all I could think about was, "How am I gonna cope? How can I live without him?" But then I reminded myself, I'll still be me. I've survived tough times before and come out better for it, and I will again.'

Bob smiled and nodded in agreement.

'The strange thing is,' I continued, 'while I was tossing and turning all night, trying to rationalise all that fear, rage and despair that was bubbling up inside me, I kept having these epiphanies, lessons I'd learned from my previous disasters. And now I feel transformed!'

He stared at me in wonder.

'I know it sounds crazy,' I said, smiling, 'but I'm almost excited about my new life. I'm even thinking of writing a book about it. Maybe I'll call it *How to Get Over Betrayal in 12 Hours*.'

Bob crooked his head and regarded me with a mix of awe and bemusement.

'You're a bloody marvel, Kat.' He paused, suddenly serious. 'But allow me to offer you a few pieces of advice. First, never say a bad word about your husband to your kids.'

I nodded in agreement.

'Second, a good divorce is when both parties are equally unhappy with the result, so stay out of court. Nobody but the lawyers will win.'

I mock-saluted and replied, 'Yes sir!' Then, I pointed to the floor and in an authoritative voice commanded, 'Now drop and give me 20.'

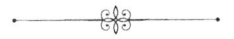

Stella was getting up for breakfast as I finished my session with Bob. There was no point in keeping anything a secret from her. I gave the local rumour mill until lunchtime before our dirty laundry was aired. Delivering this news to my baby girl was going to hurt my heart more than anything I'd ever had to do. How does someone tell their child their dad is leaving, that life as they've known it will be changing radically? For me, the answer was clear: without fuss, without drama and without victimhood or fear.

'Honey,' I began, 'Dad has a new partner. He's going to be with Tahlia now, which is great because she's really nice.' I ended the statement with what I hoped was cheerful enthusiasm.

Okay, it wasn't even close to an inspiring, overtime Super Bowl speech, but I was running on adrenaline and no sleep. More importantly, I was trying not to spin this into a 'bad news story', my theory being that bad news repeated ad nauseam would only lead to a world of endless bad news, like a sneaky social algorithm on Facebook. Because, before you realised it, your world would be full of nothing but conspiracy theories and cat videos. If I could keep my response light and positive, if I could focus on the opportunities rather than the losses, I could set the tone for how Stella and the rest of the kids responded to their new reality. Stella seemed a little perplexed as she rubbed her eyes, trying to process the information I'd just fed her.

'Wait, uh, what?'

'All will be okay my darling, no need to stress. Now, how would you like your eggs? Scrambled or fried?'

One kid down, two to go. My favourite prayer came to mind: God, grant me the serenity to accept the things I cannot change, the courage to change the things I can, and the wisdom to know the difference. My older boys were scheduled to arrive home from boarding school on the weekend, so I figured I would wait and tell them then. After Stella left for school I called my father—aka the King. His majesty had long since forbidden divorce in our family. I dreaded having to tell him his beloved son-in-law was now an out-law.

I swallowed a courage pill and announced as upbeat as I could muster, 'Dad, I'm going to be a divorcée.'

I vowed years ago to do my best to not be the cause of any more grey hairs for my dad. But somehow I still managed it. I summarised the events of the past 24 hours, starting with the fact I'd initially wanted to disappear into a bottle of wine and ending with how I'd transformed this crisis into an opportunity. By the time I said goodbye, Dad's initial shock had worn off and his understanding of my mindset was much clearer, aided by the fact he was well aware of my life history and dedication to Buddhist philosophy.

For the rest of the morning, I continued monitoring my thoughts like a lion, pouncing on anything even remotely fatalistic. Whenever I noticed my mind beginning to spiral into a vortex of fear, anger or resentment I told myself, 'Stop! Don't believe that thought! Right now, at this very moment, everything in your life is fine.' I knew I'd be a goner the moment I allowed feelings of dread, fear or desperation to sink their teeth into me. But I sure as hell went through a few dozen rounds of 'Chillax, it's going to be okay' trying not to fall off the cliff.

As promised, my mother-in-law arrived later that morning and enveloped me in an extra-tight hug, assuring me I was loved and would always be family. I'd long since forgiven her, having realised how hard it must have been for her to be placed in such a compromising position. Rosie's kind and compassionate ways of dealing with life's trials and tribulations never ceased to amaze me. She always knew what to say and when to say it. I had long ago anointed her the Dalai Lama of Jrudgerie.

By late afternoon I was starting to get a handle on how to keep my mind at peace. Stella and I drove to the man-made lake near my house where I'd planned to train with a friend for an upcoming four-day kayak race. Our timing was extraordinary. As we pulled up, there *she* was, walking her dog around the lake.

Tahlia.

We met head-on, like two out-of-control cars destined to crash. My heart beat rapidly. What the hell? Was the universe trying to test me? Stella looked at me nervously.

'Hey Stella, do you reckon I should punch her out?'

Poor Stella was horrified. 'No Mum!'

'I'm kidding,' I laughed, then lowered my window.

Tahlia approached us tentatively, clearly feeling just as awkward and uncomfortable as I was. She put on her best game face and attempted a smile.

'Should we go for a walk?'

I nodded towards the lake. 'I'd like to, but I have training.'

Stella piped up, 'I'll come with you Tahlia.' She looked to me for approval.

So here was my test. I hesitated then smiled. 'Of course.'

She jumped out of the car to play with Tahlia's dog, Barky, who she loved to death. I could never quite comprehend why. He barked incessantly and ate his own faeces for God's sake!

Tahlia took a deep breath. 'Um, Friday night Trev and I thought we'd have a barbecue tea here at the lake with the kids and maybe his parents. Would you like to join us?'

'Ah hell, why not.' It wasn't like things could get any weirder. 'I'll bring a salad.'

Tahlia was visibly relieved. I doubted she imagined our first encounter would end up being so bizarrely normal.

'Great! See you then.' She gave Barky a firm tug and made a swift departure.

I watched from behind my steering wheel as my daughter happily trotted off with my husband's new girlfriend and her dog. A mixture of sadness and acceptance swept over me. I found myself ruminating over the new trajectory my life had suddenly taken. It was truly bizarre; I felt like I'd suddenly been thrust into an episode of *The Twilight Zone* where another woman had taken over my body and my life and assumed my identity, leaving me scrambling around for a new one. I just hoped it wasn't one of those episodes where I got completely erased. What if my kids just ignored me and hung out with their less strict, 'fun' dad and his cool girlfriend while I sat at home knitting scratchy wool sweaters?

I walked to the lake's edge, composed myself and sank into the front seat of the waiting double kayak. Cindy, my teammate, was positioned in the back, ready to go. As we paddled into the calm waters, I filled her in on the last 24 hours, nodding in Stella and Tahlia's direction. Cindy was aghast.

'Does Stella know?'

'I told her this morning.'

'And you've got no problem with them hanging out together?'

I explained how I'd concluded that the best thing for me—for all of us—was to embrace our newly extended family and move on. Cindy shook her head in disbelief and powered forward with her paddle.

'I'm finding it hard to comprehend how your brain works.'

The water on the lake was mirror-like, perfectly reflecting my inner calm back at me. I felt at peace as my kayak blade cut through its surface in time with Cindy's.

'You know, Cindy, strange as it sounds, I really like Tahlia, and so do the kids. What kind of person would I be if I expected Stella and the boys to hate her because she's doing their dad? How would that benefit any of us?'

Cindy stopped paddling.

'Are you insane?'

'No. Not at all. I've just decided to take the path of love and forgiveness.'

Cindy was speechless for a few moments. We watched Stella throw a stick for Tahlia's dog.

'Are you *really* okay?'

I sighed and smiled. 'I am. Not being an emotional mess is invigorating.'

We started paddling again, syncing into an easy rhythm.

'The thing is, there's absolutely nothing I can do to change any of this, so I've decided to be happy about it.'

I could sense she was still dubious.

'Look, the two of them are in love—or maybe it's lust, I don't know—but what I do know and can't change is the fact my marriage is over.'

'Wow,' exclaimed Cindy. 'Do you mind if I hate them for you?'

'Thoughtful, Cind, but unnecessary. I'm choosing to be happy for them. I'm doing a Kat-flip, a mental righting reflex. It's far more constructive. I'm even thinking about writing a book about the process, a kind of survival manual for the soul.'

We continued to paddle in wide circles around the lake, smiling and waving at Stella and Tahlia each time we glided past.

'This is really awkward,' Cindy whispered under her breath.

'I know, it's bloody hard, but I'm hoping it'll get easier,' I whispered back.

And by our third lap around the lake, it did.

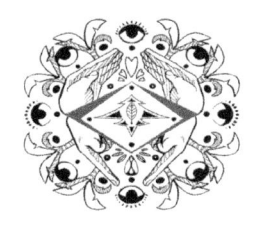

CHAPTER THREE
12 Principles for a Happier Life

I love those who can smile in trouble, who can gather strength from distress, and grow brave by reflection. 'Tis the business of little minds to shrink, but they whose heart is firm, and whose conscience approves their conduct, will pursue their principles unto death.
~ Leonardo da Vinci

I stared at the looming blank page of the journal in front of me. It was both terrifying and thrilling. I was sitting at the desk in my office, contemplating the enormity of the task that lay in front of me. Earlier, Stella and I had dined on leftover chicken cooked by Trevor the night before—thanks Trev—but now I was alone with my thoughts.

I wrote out the title across the top of the page: *How to Get Over Betrayal in 12 Hours*. There, at least I'd started. It wasn't that I couldn't write. I mean I'd written several health and fitness articles over the years, but writing an entire book, wow, that was a whole different kettle of fish. Nonetheless, I felt compelled. If

I could ease the suffering of just one other person who found themselves in a similar situation to mine, it would be a worthwhile endeavour. I flashed back to the chicken bone hitting the bedroom wall. Betrayal sucked! But suffering could be overcome with wisdom and knowledge. Like a greasy chicken stain, it could be wiped off the whiteboard of life with focused intention and effort.

So how best to explain my epiphanies, my rationalisations, and convey a lifetime of dealing with tragedies into words that made sense, that encapsulated all the wisdom it took to become a master of disaster? I needed to create a set of powerful tools for people to move forward with, irrespective of their life experience. A way for them to awaken their innate superpowers and form a new perspective to extract meaning and growth from adversity. A way to face the inevitable setbacks down the road with confidence and courage. Because the one thing I knew with absolute conviction was that once you committed to making that mental flip in perception, once you viewed betrayal through the rose-coloured lenses of karma, compassion and empathy, there was no turning back. I replayed the previous night in my head and began jotting down the realisations as they came to mind.

Master Your Thoughts
I ultimately have control over the thoughts I choose to believe in. So I need to take control of my destructive inner critic and focus on the stories that will create a better version of myself and the world I want to experience. No one can hurt me as much as I can hurt myself.

Acknowledge Impermanence

Expecting things to remain the same is a recipe for suffering. Everyone and everything has a use-by date—the good times, the bad times, relationships, health, jobs, friendships, identities, marriage...life. I need to accept that while endings can be painful, they can also create space for new beginnings.

Find a Purpose in the Pain

I can choose to let my darkest hours empower me or embitter me. So why not let pain be a catalyst for my greatest change and growth? The trick is to transform it into something more purposeful—a life lesson, an opportunity to move forward in a new direction, a chance to build resilience and push past my perceived limits.

Respond With Radical Acceptance

The more I try to deny or escape a painful reality, the more entangled I become in the tentacles of its embrace. So if it's like this now, I need to ask myself, what is my wisest response for my present and future happiness? I need to be radical with my acceptance. I control how long I suffer, no one else!

Unleash the Power of Perception

My perceptions shape my reality. When I change my perception, I can change how I experience the world and this in turn changes me. Problems no longer remain problems if I can flip my perception and see them as a series of unfolding life lessons.

Let Go of Unhealthy Attachments

Ignorantly attaching to negative thoughts, unhealthy beliefs and destructive behaviours destroys happiness. I need to acknowledge that the things I love and cherish will change and are always changing, along with my identity and my place in the world. So why isn't now the perfect time to let go of what's no longer serving me?

Enable Empathy and Compassion

Empathy and compassion help transform suffering into a shared experience. My suffering is not special or unique, but it does allow me to relate and empathise with others who've been through something similar.

Embrace Radical Forgiveness

To be radical with my forgiveness I need to go all in and understand it's not giving up or giving in but an unconditional act of great strength. Forgiveness isn't something I primarily need to do for others, but it is the best thing I can do for myself. It clears out space in the heart and mind for future peace and happiness.

Use Gratitude as a Game Changer

An attitude of gratitude silences the voices of complaint, negativity and depression in my head. When I stop focusing on what's going wrong and start focusing on what's going right then I am reminded of all of my abundance and everything I have to be thankful for.

Take Action to Create Better Karma
Karma is a mirror, reflecting my past actions back at me. Cause and effect, action and reaction. If I want to own it rather than be a victim of it, I need to ask what role I've played in creating the conditions for my present reality. And then look at planting better karmic seeds!

Cast Off the Mantle of Victimhood
My happiness is no one else's responsibility, my suffering is no one else's fault. I am equally the creator of my detonators and the master of my disasters. I need to ditch the blame game, the judgemental attitude and the pity parties and claim back my power.

Become a Maestro of Manifestation
THINK, SPEAK, ACT and BE what I want my future world to look like. Maintain clarity and conviction around what I actually want to cultivate and take action in this present moment to make it happen.

I stopped writing and looked over my work. It was a good start. A wave of cathartic joy washed over me. *Keep going Kitty, you can do this!* Controlling the mind, embracing impermanence, turning pain into strength—these were the principles on which I'd built my house of knowledge and wisdom. I thought back to my inauspicious birth, my father's tough love, my struggles and conquests, knowing they had prepared me in some way for the suffering and disasters to come. Was it too much of a stretch to believe they'd also been leading me to this point, where I could write this book and help others? Why else would God, the Universe, fate—call it what you will—put me through so much agony? Because even in my tenderest years I found myself enduring the type of pain that either crushes you or forces you to rise from the ashes.

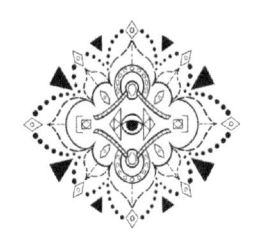

CHAPTER FOUR
The Child Who Should Have Been Drowned at Birth

Give me a child until he is seven, and I will show you the man.
~ Aristotle

For as long as I can remember I've yearned for adventure. There was always an itch I couldn't scratch, a hole in my soul, a higher goal to achieve. The grass on the other side was always greener, the rut always deeper. Good or bad, it didn't matter to me. I wanted something more, something different. Not surprisingly, agitation was my shadow, leaving me wondering if what I had would ever be enough. For most of my life, the notion of peace and contentment eluded me.

To understand the end, sometimes you need to start at the beginning.

I entered the world in a Toronto hospital on a cold and rainy autumn day. It was 1972, and bell bottoms and wide-collared shirts were still in vogue. According to my dry-humoured, grimly hilarious, sports-mad father, my early arrival couldn't have been timed more poorly. It heralded the beginning of a chain of events that proved to be a nightmare for him. Mum went into labour during the third game of the Canada-vs-Russia hockey series, the ultimate hockey event of the year for Canadian hockey fans. Dad had no choice but to miss the entire third period of the game and was not impressed that I stubbornly refused to come out for another 30 hours. This was highly uncharacteristic of me—normally I would have leapt at the opportunity for a new experience. Dad paced and waited, waited and paced. Thanks to his classically English upbringing, the very idea of being present in the same room as the birth was barbaric. The doctor soon lost patience, clamped forceps around my delicate skull and unceremoniously yanked me out of my mother's womb like the cork from an old bottle of French red. I carry the scar on the back of my head to this day.

My mother endured the labour and birth stoically. Thankfully she was accustomed to stoicism, having arrived in Canada as a refugee with her family only a few years earlier. They were fleeing Russia's attempt to crush a mass uprising in their native Czechoslovakia. Mum was petite and beautiful. She had soft, chocolate-coloured eyes and long, silky black hair that she wore in a high ponytail. She spoke and understood English well, but her accent sometimes made it difficult for others to understand what she was saying. Mum bestowed me with the middle name Samantha, a homage to the episodes of *Bewitched* that had taught her most of her English. The hospital set our discharge date for a few days later. It just happened to coincide with the final game of the Canada–Russia hockey series. Dad was horrified all over again. Mum thought it best for all concerned to put off returning home with me until the next day so he could watch the final game in peace. Canada won. He was ecstatic. The world was saved.

However, the inconvenience of my premature arrival continued to haunt poor Dad. A month still remained on their lease at the adults-only apartment building where they lived, so they had no choice but to smuggle me in. Their mission during the first month of my life was to keep me under the radar of the superintendent. I screamed all night, every night, unless I was the babe in arms being walked up and down the hallway. How the superintendent never found out was a miracle. I was the perfect trifecta of disasters—early, noisy and inconsiderate of major sports events—resulting in my father jokingly referring to me as 'the child I should've drowned at birth'. At least I thought he was joking.

Right before Dad reached the end of his tether, the lease expired and we moved into a kid-friendly bungalow just in time for my sister's birth. Story of my life. Here I was, barely a year old and already cast as the rebel of the family. Mum wanted to call my sister Endora, which was Samantha's mother's name on *Bewitched*, but Dad put his foot down. She ended up a Wendy instead. My sis was the perfect baby, and nothing much has changed since.

Although Dad claimed to be unbiased when it came to his kids, he would often declare, 'I love all of you kids the same, but Wendy is just the best.' We unanimously agreed. Wendy hated the title, which only cemented the fact that she was and still is 'the best'. Shortly after Wendy, my brother Martin arrived. And then in quick succession came my next two sisters, Caroline and Tracy. They were both born talking and we are still waiting for them to stop. Martin, on the other hand, was a quiet child. Perhaps being born smack in the middle of four talkative sisters meant he never really had a chance to express his opinion or get a word in. He was nearly four before he spoke.

There was only one way to describe our home life in the ensuing years: chaotic. By the time the final two arrived, there were seven of us crammed into the miniature three-bedroom bungalow. Fights erupted constantly, especially over things like the last Oreo, cheap cereal box toys and whether we'd watch *The Flintstones* or *The Brady Bunch*. We slept on top of each other in space-saving Scandinavian-designed bunk beds. Occasionally there were attempted hostile takeovers of the top bunk, but my iron will, tenacity and power of persuasion meant I always won the battles. I might have made a good lawyer had it not been for my laissez-faire attitude towards schooling.

At bedtime every night Dad would read Enid Blyton stories, usually *The Famous Five*, followed by some standard Catholic prayers. This instilled a lifelong passion for books in all of us—and maybe a sense of adventure in me—and helped us bond together as a family. To this day, my siblings and I remain very close, although I still personally harbour my fair share of

Catholic guilt thanks to those childhood prayers reminding me that an all-knowing, all-seeing God is constantly watching over me, passing judgement.

Like our house, our neighbourhood also overflowed with kids. There was a constant stream of children flowing in and out our front door. Being constantly surrounded by siblings, friends and family provided me with a strong sense of belonging. Although there were times I yearned for some time and space to myself, the funny thing was, on the rare occasions I actually achieved this, I immediately started to feel lonely and restless. This discomfort with loneliness stuck with me well into my adult life.

In the summer road hockey and hide-and-seek consumed our free time, while in the winter it centred around tobogganing and building igloos. Sometimes we'd shovel a big pile of snow behind my parents' car and spend hours sliding from the roof down the back windscreen to land in it. I remember many days Mum running late to pick up Dad from the train because she'd been forced to frantically dig out the car from the snowbank we'd created. The only two hard and fast rules we had to abide by while playing outside were to stay within the boundaries of the neighbourhood and head home when the streetlights came on. Of course, during the shorter, colder months that meant most of the gang would congregate at our place afterwards for hot chocolate and couch jumping before Dad got home from work. It was bedlam.

Being the eldest of the tribe, I was always being asked by my mother to help look after the kids. I was always being shoved into the 'responsible leadership' role. Looking back, it's hard to say what moulded my personality more: my inherent restlessness and my stubborn nature or being responsible for four younger brothers and sisters from an early age. Either way, it resulted in me swearing black and blue I'd never have any children of my own. I often wondered, why are there so many of us? Why couldn't my parents just have been happy with one or two kids? Could they not have simply loved me more? I daydreamed about what it would be like to have my mother's undivided attention, even for a mere five minutes.

The upshot was, I was expected to be a leader, but instead I rebelled and became the black sheep of the family. I took out my frustrations and my unbridled energy on those around me by inflicting various misdemeanours and misadventures on friends and family. Some of these crossed the line into 'danger' territory, but the way I figured it, it was all just part of the fun. How I managed to survive my childhood without injuring myself or others in any serious way, was something of a minor miracle.

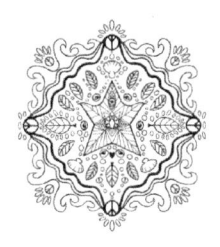

CHAPTER FIVE
Affection Is Reserved for the Italians

Don't be unhappy about someone else's happiness...it's not your loss.
~ Brian Finnerty (aka Dad)

What is love? For some people it's hugs, cuddles and words of affection. For our family, love was shown more pragmatically through cooking, cleaning and doing what you were told. Being upset or emotional was seen as a weakness, something to be overcome, banished, conquered. Affection was a cuff on the cheek or a ruffle of the hair. Dad stated categorically that open displays of affection were reserved for other cultures, like the Italians.

Some of my dad's favourite expressions were 'Stop crying or I'll give you something to cry about' and 'Life's not fair, get over it.' This concept of life not playing fair was drummed into me from an early age, along with the idea that to 'get over it' I had to be grateful for what I had, stop complaining about what I didn't have and strive to do my best without expecting constant rewards. If we complained about a sore ear, his remedy was as harsh as it was simple: 'Come here and I'll chop it off for you.'

This stoic training in how to quickly overcome challenges without wallowing in emotions had several advantages. It helped me cope more pragmatically with my many childhood disasters, it taught me how to short-cut my suffering and it alerted me to the fact that the consumerist culture I was growing up in was selling me a false dream: this idea that I deserved better, that the key to happiness lay in satisfying my wants and desires, and that if I worked hard enough, made all the right decisions and looked after number one then life would reward me with happiness and 'play fair'. I knew better from my family life.

Despite his seemingly harsh exterior and archaic worldviews, our father was kind and loving in his own unique way. If we did a good job, he might say something distinctly understated and British like, 'Well that wasn't nearly as bad as it could have been.' He had his own manual for life and a strict set of rules, which we respected. If he was able to rationalise something as right, it didn't matter what anyone else or society thought. He was, and still is, a serial non-conformist who regularly exclaims, 'Things will change when I am king.' To be honest, I think there's a lot of Dad in me as well.

Mum, on the other hand, was in love with being a mum. She wanted to fill the house with kids and happiness, and she succeeded. Everyone who came to our home was treated as part of the family, even though many of our friends struggled at times to understand Mum's strongly accented English. When she asked our friends what they wanted in their sandwich for lunch, they would look quizzically at us for a translation.

'Hum? U vant hum?' No answer.

'I said, do u vant hum?' she would shout, hoping the louder she spoke, the more likely she'd be understood.

'Ham!' we would eventually burst out through fits of laughter.

Having five kids plus a never-ending assortment of friends meant Mum didn't have much time to herself, although she did manage to steal away once a week to an aerobics class. One day when she came home with chocolate on her chin, she confessed to me she'd stayed near the back of the class with her friend so they could sneak out early for ice cream.

'Life, my darlink, es meant to be a pervect balans between pleasure und pain.'

I soaked up this little gem of wisdom, and it's been my go-to mantra ever since. Despite having to constantly translate Mum's accent to friends, I never learnt to speak Czech even though she spoke it with her family and friends. She preferred not having us privy to her every conversation. The only word I ever learnt was *ahoj*, which means 'hello'.

Thanks to our parents' respective upbringings—Dad toughing it out during the post-war years in England, Mum living hard in an Eastern Bloc Communist country—frugality was drummed into us on a daily basis. If there was something we wanted but didn't need, there was a good chance we went without it. Dad made it clear to us at an early age that having an innate sense of entitlement was selfishness in disguise and would only lead to future pain and suffering. This 'waste not, want not' attitude was ingrained into all of us kids and even to this day, I abhor throwing food away or spending money frivolously. I guess I could have chosen to see my father's strict rules and no-nonsense attitude towards emotional weakness as harsh and restrictive. But instead, I embraced it and used it as a way to infuse grit into every aspect of my life.

Our childhood wasn't all coupon-cutting and discipline, however. There were plenty of fun times, games and laughter as well. I remember getting up at 6 a.m. with Mum and joining her for her daily morning TV workout routine with Richard Simmons. I wore a headband and legwarmers and looked like a miniature Jane Fonda. And then there were the days Mum would pile all five of us into the car extra early to go pick up Dad from the train station. Why early? Because the parking lot at the station had a rise in it that acted like a giant skateboard ramp. Mum would line up the car then yell at us to hang on as she floored it. We'd hit the edge and our little bodies would launch off the seats, free of the constraints of gravity or seatbelts, suspended between earth and sky, or at least leather and vinyl, until we landed with a bounce on the other side, prompting us to yell, 'Again, again!' And to our joy, she would circle the car around and hit it a few more times, like a female Evil Knievel chasing the thrill of the ride.

Our car-jumping adventures provided me with a rare glimpse into the hidden side of my mum, the side that was wild, free and unrestrained. I remember thinking, *I wanna be like that, I wanna be someone who can throw caution to the wind and live life as if there is no tomorrow.* I hoped that this irrepressible and beautiful side of Mum existed somewhere inside me too, forever protecting me from a life of monotony and boredom.

Mum's car jumping days were complimented by more sedate family activities like jigsaw puzzles. And man, did we do loads of them! It was one of the reasons we rarely ate at the formal dining table. We'd all gather round and spend hours trying to complete them, cheering and clapping with glee when we'd finally slot the last piece into place. I learnt quickly that every piece of a puzzle, no matter how difficult to figure out, eventually contributes to the bigger picture and has its place and purpose. And I learnt to replace my 'furiousity' with curiosity and my irritation with conciliation. It was a lightbulb moment for me, the idea that something so simple as a puzzle could help me navigate life by teaching me not to overreact in anger when things didn't go my way.

The other magical thing about our family puzzles were that they transcended age, cultures and language, which proved to be very handy in a half-Czech, half-British household. As children, we weren't cognisant of the different cultures in our home. It was normal to have our paternal grandparents visit us on Fridays, bringing homemade apple pies, white bread rolls and ham, while on Saturdays our maternal grandparents showed up with dark rye, matzo ball soup and Hungarian salami.

Dad's Catholic upbringing meant that every Sunday, without fail, we went to church at St. Martin de Porres. This was followed by exhaustively boring Sunday school. We were convinced that whoever came up with 'school' on a weekend should be sacked. Dad, however, was insistent that our young minds be exposed to the morality encompassed within his faith. I found the Bible stories far-fetched, but some of the morals did sink in and I especially appreciated the concept that no matter how badly you sinned, you could still be forgiven if you simply repented at the end and threw yourself at the mercy of God. This aligned perfectly with my way of doing life.

Mum never came with us to church: rather she claimed the time as her opportunity to do the weekly grocery shop without five kids pestering her to buy the box of cereal with the best toy inside. There was, however, one saving grace to our Sunday morning rituals and that was lunch at McDonald's. It was the ultimate bribe for having to endure the boredom of a whole morning's religious education.

Our only other 'gourmet' treat was a mid-week family outing to the nearby bakery for a six-pack of doughnuts. Dad would order his premium pastry, an enormous éclair stuffed with real whipped cream and topped with chocolate, which left the budget half-dozen to be divided among the rest of us. Mum was forever on a diet, so her doughnut was given to Martin, perhaps as a peace offering for having to endure the torments of four sisters.

One day I bravely lodged a complaint about the unfairness of the doughnut deal. My dad immediately took my doughnut, gave it to Martin and, with the burning tip of his cigarette waving in front of my face, stated, 'Never be unhappy about somebody else's happiness.' Seconds later he took all three doughnuts from my smirking brother's hands and gave them to my sisters. 'And you son, don't you be happy about your sister's unhappiness.' And there it was, profound life lessons demonstrated by deep-fried dough.

This effectively put an end to the doughnut discord and took care of any future sense of entitlement in our household. To this day I try to be happy about everyone else's happiness knowing that my happiness doesn't result from me getting a better deal but from everyone getting a better deal! And I try not to complain about what I haven't got and instead do my best to notice and be grateful for what I have got. What you covet can be taken away in a puff of smoke.

Being restricted to a single doughnut once a week may have seemed like cruel and unusual punishment for any kid, but for me it was a necessity. I was hyperactive and didn't need the extra sugar hit. I was the child who couldn't sit still, who had boundless energy, who was curious, outgoing, mischievous and constantly on the lookout for trouble or the next wild adventure. I got a kick out of taking risks and I assumed everyone else did too.

My habit of wandering off and dragging others with me on clandestine adventures earned me the nickname 'The Happy Wanderer'. My sister Wendy, for example, was quiet and shy. I saw this as a character flaw she needed help to overcome. At the tender age of three, I pushed her into an empty elevator in a 20-story building and hit the close button so she could build up some much needed courage. And during an enforced babysitting gig of my sister Tracy, I tied her to the dining table, then left her there while I went to hang out at a friend's house nearby. My friend's parents, on hearing of my exploits, sent me straight back home to untie her even though I explained I'd sensibly left the TV on for her so she wouldn't get bored. My little brother Martin didn't escape my attention either. I would convince him to ride his bike with me to the treacherous cliffs of the Scarborough Bluffs and then, once there, jump on the edge of the cliff to try and create a rockslide all the way down into Lake Ontario.

But by far my most harrowing adventure occurred with one of my best friends, Karen, at the 'forbidden forest', a steep ravine a few blocks from my house. It was off limits thanks to it being a hangout for local potheads. But because it was winter, even the potheads had seemingly given up toking in the great outdoors in exchange for some indoor comfort and warmth. So I dragged Karen along with me for some fun. The path we walked on towards the ravine was covered in ice. We navigated forward by skating and sliding from one bare tree trunk to the next. To the side of us was a steep cliff covered with vegetation sloped down to a rocky creek.

Without warning one of the saplings snapped at the base and both of us skidded off the edge and began tumbling down the cliff face into the ravine. The only thing that saved us from plummeting straight to the bottom was a half-fallen tree trunk. We clung to it as if our lives depended on it, which they probably did, and screamed for help. Eventually, a man came out of a nearby house, threw us a rope and hauled us up. I thought this was a grand adventure. Karen, on the other hand, was left scarred for life and her figure skating career ended not long after that fateful day.

Sadly, my pain-free existence was fast coming to an end. The first of my childhood disasters was rapidly approaching, and I would soon discover that pleasure and pain were flipsides of the same coin. Ironically, the danger would emanate not from my interactions with the outside world, but from the world within.

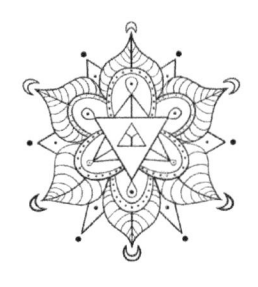

CHAPTER SIX
The Flipside of Pleasure Is Pain

*You never know how strong you are
until being strong is your only choice.
- Bob Marley*

I was only six years old when I began to suffer from horrific migraines, inherited from Dad's side of the family. It's hard to find words to describe the intensity of the pain I endured because, unlike a grazed knee or a bumped elbow, it was difficult to disassociate my mind from the injury. Migraines exploded inside my head like fireworks. They'd strike fast and mercilessly, always following the same pattern. My vision would blur, then light would begin to hurt my eyes and I'd throw up, after which my head would start pounding like a kettledrum.

Mum tried everything to help me. She took me to our GP, and when that didn't work, she took me to paediatricians, chiropractors, psychologists, podiatrists, optometrists, herbalists, and nutritionists. I had X-rays, CAT scans, manipulations, eye tests. Mum's quest was relentless, her mission was to find out why my migraines were happening and how we could stop them.

The result of all this intensive investigation was the identification of specific triggers that seemed to bring on the migraines. For example, red food dye hit the mark every time: taco seasoning, red Smarties, my favourite red liquorice, Twizzlers, plus so many of the foods that brought me pleasure in life, like chocolate and cheese. Consuming any of them ended in pain. The good news was at least I could avoid eating the wrong foods. What I found much harder to deal with were the emotional triggers.

Getting really excited about something, like the last day of school or an excursion to a theme park or birthday parties or Christmas, was sure to bring on another life-interrupting migraine. One doctor prescribed a strong drug to counteract this, but it had to be taken just as the migraine was forming. If I took the pill as soon as I noticed my vision going or light beginning to hurt, I could avoid a full-blown attack. Great idea in theory. But because the migraines generally hit when I was about to do something exciting and fun, I often pretended I was fine and would studiously ignore the developing symptoms. Invariably I'd end up vomiting and with an excruciating headache, leaving my parents shaking their heads in frustration as they scrubbed the vomit off someone's floor.

The pain during these episodes was intense. It felt like an enraged dragon breathing fire in my head. It didn't matter where I was or what I was doing at the time. I'd immediately have to find a dark place, lie down, try to be as still as possible, and wait for the beast in my brain to calm down. Any noise, light or movement was agony. Even at a young age, I realised if I allowed myself to get upset, if I let my fear and emotions take over, the pain would worsen dramatically.

It would have made more sense to prevent the pain in the first place, but I always pushed the envelope, thinking, 'Maybe this time it'll be okay. Maybe this time I won't ruin someone's carpet or a family day at the waterpark.' I refused to let the inevitable be a threat or the fear of the ensuing pain rule my life. I figured out the best way to survive the worst of my migraines was to modify my perceptions. All I had to do was allow my thoughts to focus on a slow breath and visualise a dim, healing light wrapping itself around my head and absorbing the pain. With every exhale I released the pain into the light. I didn't know it then, but I was practising a form of meditation.

This concept helped me through 12 long years of excruciating migraines, which inexplicably stopped when I was 18, but my meditations and ability to control and manage pain would become a cornerstone of my yoga and Buddhist training later in life. There was, however, one incident from which even my budding meditation skills couldn't save me.

When I was ten, my great-aunt Kath from California visited our house in Toronto. She and Uncle Herbie parked their enormous Winnebago out front, taking up nearly the entire length of our curb. Aunt Kath was always fashionably dressed—not great-aunt style, but trendy and cool. She was my idol and the best part was, she adored me as well. She loved her Tanqueray gin, and the party started as soon as the bottle was cracked. During one of these parties, I was struck down with yet another migraine and ended up vomiting uncontrollably, nearly blinded by the pain.

My great-aunt was well aware of what I was going through, having personally known the pain of migraines, but she exclaimed to my mother she'd never seen a young child suffer such terrible pain. Having had too much to drink and being far more assertive than when sober, she was adamant I needed hospitalisation and attempted to load me into the Winnebago. Mum, thankfully, insisted we take the car and that she would drive.

I'll never forget being forced out of my bed, where I could be still and allow my mind to go someplace else, and into the back of that car. Every bump on the road, every movement, every sound was agony as my mind erupted in geysers of pain. At the hospital, I was forced to lie under bright, fluorescent lights on a hard bed. All I wanted to do was go home, curl up in a dark place and suffer in peace rather than lying exposed in an indiscreet hospital gown, vomiting my guts out.

After what seemed like an eternity, a tall, surly nurse with a pinched nose and round glasses showed up to take my blood. She towered over me, repeatedly jabbing a needle into my tiny arm to find a vein. It was awful. I closed my eyes and did my best to remove myself from the situation. I didn't shed a tear. I was an expert on pain and knew that crying wouldn't help. In fact, being emotional would have made it far worse. My father's 'tough love' proved to be a blessing. But the experience did instill in me a fear of needles, and to this day I avoid them like cats avoid swimming.

I could tell my mother was horrified at the nurse's actions, but she was too intimidated to speak up. Aunt Kath was passed out in a chair, so she was no help either. When Nurse Frankenstein noticed I'd vomited up all previous attempts at oral pain relief, she ordered me to roll over, face the wall and curl into a ball. I wondered why but my head was still pounding, and I was too weak to speak. To my horror, she told me to pull down my underpants. I was a modest child, and this was beyond embarrassing for me.

The next thing I knew, a suppository had been shoved up where the sun never shines. I was shocked. I couldn't believe the nurse had just violated me in that way. The suppository did work, but I was left traumatised. At some point I finally stopped vomiting, my migraine receded and I once again joined the land of the living. Another 30 years would pass before I would find myself in a similar position, curled up in a hospital bed in a foetal position, feeling utterly powerless. Only this time the bed was in Greece, and the needle being repeatedly stabbed into me wasn't into my arm but into my spinal cord. It nearly killed me.

Looking back, I believe my migraine experience helped me become more resilient and contributed to me having an inordinately high pain threshold. I now rarely shed tears when I'm experiencing serious pain, either physically or emotionally. In fact, it was pivotal in helping me weather the next of my childhood disasters, which proved far more devastating and painful than any of my migraines and severely tested my belief and faith in God.

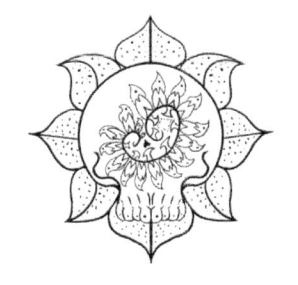

CHAPTER SEVEN
Tiny but Tuff

Some people, sweet and attractive, and strong and healthy,
happen to die young.
They are teachers in disguise teaching us about impermanence.
~ Dalai Lama XIV

I stared at the phone, willing it to ring. It was the morning of my 12th birthday. I'd awakened early, eagerly anticipating a call from my mother and was reluctant to leave for school until I had spoken to her. There was no way she could forget. Today of all days, she would surely make the effort to call me.

In the months preceding my birthday, Mum had spent considerable time away. The odd weekend she did come home, she would send us kids outside while she chatted with friends who visited the moment they heard she was home. It upset me terribly. I'd known she would be away for my birthday but thought at the very least she'd call. Dad made me go to school, and I reluctantly trudged off—one did not argue with the King—but when I arrived I was glad I had gone. My birthday was announced at assembly and the entire junior high sang 'Happy Birthday'. Friends, teachers and families I'd known for years showered me with gifts, birthday hugs and good wishes. I felt like a rock star.

By lunchtime I'd forgotten about my mother not calling, so overwhelmed was I by all the attention. The celebrations continued when I returned home that afternoon. Neighbours, my grandparents and friends crammed into our shoebox of a house, laden with brownies, strawberry shortcakes and cheesy lasagnas. By coincidence, two of my friends gave me the exact same gift—t-shirts printed with *Tiny but Tuff*. This slogan summed me up in three simple but powerful words. So many people came, all bringing gifts because they knew what I did not: that my world was about to change forever.

Dad came home just as dusk was setting in. I was on a sugar high. He called me into his bedroom. I waited with bated breath to see the wonderful birthday gift he'd brought for me. As I stood proudly in front of him, twirling around showing off my new t-shirt, I saw tears well up in his eyes. My sister Wendy, next in line for my hand-me-downs, ran in, eager to see what was coming her way. I looked at her, she looked at me, then both of us turned to look at Dad. And in that moment we both knew.

Mum was dead.

My mother had been undergoing treatment for colon cancer. Unbeknownst to me, a week before my birthday, as she was slipping in and out of a coma, she swore to my father, 'I will live until Kat's birthday. I will fight to live until that day.'

Days later we stood by Mum's graveside, throwing handfuls of dirt onto her coffin. It was a bitterly cold, rainy autumn day, much like the day on which my mother brought me into the world. Dad stood beside me, holding my hand.

'Why did she have to pick my birthday to die? It's not fair.'

'It was her gift to you,' he replied gently. 'Your mum fought to stay alive, it was an incredible testament to the strength of love and the human spirit.'

He explained that against all odds, she'd lingered in and out of a coma, refusing to die until her firstborn's birthday.

'She loved you,' Dad said. 'Don't you ever forget that.'

Then he told me something I've never forgotten:

'In our lives, nothing is permanent. Not even the people we love the most. It's terribly sad and never easy, but it is life. The intensity of the pain you're feeling right now, it will fade and eventually pass, but it's up to you to decide how long that takes.'

I felt the warmth of his hand through my coat as he squeezed my shoulder gently. 'You can think of your mother's death on your birthday as a terrible tragedy, or you can think of it as a gift. I know which one your mother would have wanted you to choose.'

Looking back now, I know Dad was right. Mum filled our lives with happiness and fun. She had a zest and passion for life, underpinned by an incredible inner strength. In addition to raising five children, she dabbled in home and car maintenance, was forever volunteering to help the local community and often drove us around the city for hours to drop off clothes and household items to newly arrived Czech refugees. She was the type of person who put others needs before her own and did this with effortless grace.

My mother was 33 when she gave birth to her last child, my sister Tracy. A few months later she went to the doctor for persistent stomach pain. Initially, the doctor attributed the pain to the burden placed on Mum's body by multiple pregnancies over a short period of time. After a year of her repeated complaints, he sent her for a colonoscopy. Two days later she was on the operating table.

I was in sixth grade when my parents told us at dinner about Mum's tumour. Knowing as much about tumours as I did about astrophysics, this meant little to me until, one day in the school playground, the class know-it-all said, 'Your mum's got cancer.'

'She has not,' I replied indignantly. 'It's a tumour!' Rumours, I've learnt, are never far from the truth.

Operation after operation followed. Each time the surgeons cut, they took away another piece of her dignity, but despite being poisoned by chemo and burned with radiation, the one thing she did manage to keep was her beautiful black hair. Not as shiny or as thick, but it remained with her, as steadfast as her spirit.

As a last Hail Mary effort, Mum decided to enlist the help of a healer in New Brunswick whom her psychic recommended. All seven of us piled into our brand new Magic Wagon, the original mini-van featuring a sleek wooden strip down the side. Our estimated two-day road trip to the east coast took more than a week. Mum was so sick she needed to be hospitalised along the way when we reached Québec. We prayed for a miracle, but we were too young to understand how critical her situation was. Rather, we were excited by our impromptu getaway. We went on a horse-drawn carriage ride and dined on what we thought of as fine French cuisine at St-Hubert, which was actually Québécois fast food—their take on Kentucky Fried Chicken. We were stunned to discover that Dad spoke French when he ordered our chicken and asked for 'poulet'.

We finally arrived in New Brunswick after fruitless arguments as Dad tried to read the map and Mum just wanted to pull over and ask for directions. We finally found the healer's wellness centre, which turned out to be a dilapidated shack. Dad didn't say a word. He just got out of the car, lit up a smoke and shook his head. Our five little faces were pressed against the car windows as we watched Mum slowly make her way up the steps with Dad's help. For once we sat quietly in the car. My parents weren't gone long before they reappeared. Mum looked victorious. She was gripping her colostomy bag in one hand and a brown paper bag in the other. Us kids believed the paper bag contained a magic potion that would end her suffering. As Dad put the car in gear he turned and gave us a reassuring wink. Yes! Mum was going to get her life back.

That night we sat transfixed as Mum pulled the cork out of a vial of pungent, disgusting-looking gelatinous brown liquid the 'healer' had given her to drink. She was perched on the end of the bed in the motel room, surrounded by five kids, a chain-smoking husband and a swath of well-worn, emerald-green carpet. Could it be true that this disgusting potion was going to save her? She looked at us, smiled and then, with eyes closed, grimaced and swallowed it down, giving us the thumbs-up.

Everybody dies, but we never know what day that will be. I'm sure my mother thought she would live well past 37, that she would be blessed with more time. As did I. We were both wrong. My father, ever the realist, knew Mum's days were numbered, and so, when my youngest sister Tracy started her first day of kindergarten, Dad did something extraordinary. He busted Mum out of the hospital, enlisting the help of a nurse to detach her from all of the machines, and drove her to the school so she would be there to meet her baby daughter when the final bell rang.

Tracy never forgot that moment. The sheer joy of having her mother there, just like all the other children, to hug her after her first day of school remains one of her most enduring childhood memories of Mum. Afterwards, Dad drove his weak and exhausted but blissfully happy wife back to the hospital. This was the last time Mum and Tracy would see each other.

My final memory of Mum was of her lying on the couch at home after a last-ditch effort by doctors to save her. Most of her bowel had been removed by then, and earlier that day she'd received what turned out to be a near-lethal dose of chemo and radiation.

Despite being deathly ill, she was at home, doing her best to look after us. Cooking dinner for us gave her a purpose, a reason to push past the pain. As Mum stood frying schnitzel, she would frequently have to run to the bathroom to be sick, after which she would steal brief moments to lie on the couch.

My friend's family had invited me out for dinner that night. Mum begged me to stay and help her make dinner. I was only 11 at the time, ignorant of Mum's deteriorating condition. She pleaded with me not to go, but I selfishly mumbled, 'Sorry, I'll be back soon.' I clearly remember her face as I walked out the door. She was too weak to argue with me and instead turned her head away, trying to hide her sadness and pain.

She was hospitalised soon after. Despite knowing the end was close, Dad didn't take us to see her. He didn't want our last memory to be of Mum dying in a hospital bed. Mum felt the same way. That's why she'd send us away sometimes when she was at home. Dad said it was torture for her seeing her children, knowing she would soon be dead. She put up a strong front, never allowing us to witness the emotional and physical pain she was in. Together with my father, they agreed to protect us from the inevitable until it happened. They believed it was better for us to only have to deal with the pain once, when the end came.

I never saw my mother again. I never got a chance to tell her I was sorry for walking out on her that night. Thirty years after Mum's death I heard a story from my Uncle John that helped me process the shame I carried with me for so many years. He told me something that happened in her last moments.

'At one point your mum came out of her coma. I couldn't believe it. She was humming a song. I said to your dad, "She's singing!" and your dad replied quietly, "Yes, I know. She's singing 'Happy Birthday' to Kat, it's her birthday today." I thought by some miracle she might be getting better. Your dad looked exhausted, I told him to go grab a coffee, that I'd sit with her. He was gone for not more than five minutes when your mum stopped singing. I shook her gently, squeezed her hand and said, "Karla?" She had such a peaceful look on her face. It took me a few minutes to realise she wasn't breathing. She'd made it to your birthday, and I guess she was just waiting for your dad to leave so she could leave too.'

At 12 years old, my mother's death was terribly tragic, but it taught me some powerful truths. Every beginning has an end. Our joy and grief, our pleasure and pain, our health, family and friends all have expiration dates. All we really have control over is how we respond to change, to death, to the loss of something cherished. As Thich Nhat Hanh, a wise Buddhist monk once said, 'It's not impermanence that makes us suffer; what makes us suffer is wanting things to be permanent when they are not.'

These days I try to live my life as my mother did: with love, laughter, kindness, compassion and the occasional scoop of chocolate ice cream. Because in the end all you can do is live your best life knowing, like she did, that your enduring legacy, your most precious gift, is to leave behind family, friends and a community bonded together and made stronger by your love and by the knowledge that, although death is inevitable, life and love continue on.

CHAPTER EIGHT
Let Go and Let God

*Your worst enemy cannot harm you
as much as your own unguarded thoughts.
- Buddha*

I shivered beneath the eerie glow of streetlights as I peered over the concrete railing of the bridge. It was late, well past my curfew, the wind whipping savagely through the ravine. I could hear the waters of Highland Creek rushing across the rocks. I wondered if I really had the guts to climb onto the railing and jump. It occurred to me that no matter how many aspirins I swallowed or how much vodka I drank, it was still a long way down and landing on those rocks would hurt like hell. I'd just turned 16, and life was far from sweet.

Everything changed after Mum passed away, but not in the way I thought it would. It wasn't awful, just different. We were a pragmatic family with a staunchly British father, and there was no prolonged grieving period, no crying, no moping around. We carried on with life in her absence. Stiff upper lip and all that. On the one hand, it allowed us to move forward quickly, without dwelling in the past. But on the other, it felt as though Mum had been erased from our lives. One minute she was indispensable, the next she was gone forever.

A week after her death we went back to school and Dad went back to work. The Red Cross assisted by sending a housekeeper to help us during the day, although this wasn't always as useful as we'd hoped it would be. Toronto is a proudly multicultural city, so it became an amusing game to guess the nationality of the housekeeper who arrived each day. They were generally of Indian, Jamaican or African descent, and none bore the slightest resemblance to the Mary Poppins character we hoped for. Tracy, only four at the time, found the situation particularly confusing. It must have been hard for her to comprehend why every day, instead of her mum, there was someone new looking after her who could barely understand what she was saying. As for the reigning king of the household, Dad struggled mightily with dinner times. He considered garlic a 'foreign' food and had long banned exotic spices from our house. Now, we often sat down to meals that were far outside our comfort zone and bore little resemblance to a 'proper' English meal. Dad would insist we eat everything on our plates even while his remained noticeably untouched.

Dad might have starved if not for the arrival of a Scottish housekeeper named Sheila. She possessed a bland palate like my father, and her cooking skills were based squarely in the English culinary camp. She spoke with a thick Scottish accent and had five grown-up children of her own, so she was no stranger to the chaos of a tribe of kids. After eating her rice pudding, Dad hired her on the spot as our full-time housekeeper. Sheila looked after my younger siblings. She cooked, cleaned and did the laundry, but as good as she was at filling the void Mum had left, she was no substitute for our mother emotionally. At the end of the day, we were just a job to her. We weren't her family, and I, for one, would have run a mile before revealing my innermost feelings to her.

Puberty is a challenge at the best of times, but without Mum around I was having to navigate the whole messy process mostly by myself. I didn't like talking to others about personal matters and certainly didn't feel comfortable asking Dad to throw a pack of pads into the weekly grocery shop. I was starting to care about what I looked like, wanting to cover up pimples with makeup, wear trendy clothes and have my hair permed. The only way to accomplish all this was to become independent and financially secure, and so step one was to get a job. From the age of 13, I made it my mission to be continuously employed. I usually worked numerous jobs at once—babysitter, summer camp counsellor, checkout chick, fish and chip shop potato peeler, cleaner at the mall—you name it, I did it. I loved working, but I loved the financial freedom and sense of purpose it gave me even more. My wages meant I could now purchase the clothes I wanted, like trendy Gloria Vanderbilt jeans, Playtex bras with matching undies and Benetton polos. Dad often reminded us, 'I will buy you anything you need, not everything you want,' so if I wanted something special I had to procure it myself. This idea of being financially independent has since become a mainstay in my life, and I have never gone without. Good thing I was born and bred to be happy with the basics.

At the time, my two best friends were Anna and Charmaine. We'd known each other since kindergarten. Charmaine was an only child, tall, blonde, skinny and stylish, while Anna was short, chubby and bubbly. I was the mousey one in the middle. Anna had a brother named Tim who was three years older than us. I loved spending time with Charmaine, Anna and their families. Compared to my place, their homes were oases of calm. Anna and Charmaine had their own rooms, a constant supply of good junk food, and when I hung out with them I was free of my responsibilities. Most importantly, I felt cared for, nurtured and supported. Their mothers would take me shopping and recount to me stories of my own mother, which helped me keep her memories alive. And then everything changed two years later.

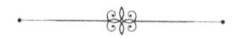

The catalyst was when we moved into a bigger house in another neighbourhood. Although I luxuriated in having a huge bedroom all to myself, it also meant a new school for me. And due to the tyranny of distance, I could no longer see Anna, Charmaine and their families on a daily basis. I was forced to start from scratch and make new friends and connections. I lost my wing-girls, my support network and the conversations about my Mum. Then Tim decided to declare his undying love for me. He was 18 at the time, had his own wheels—well, his parents' Chevy—and he visited me regularly. I thought of him as a big brother. Initially, I was repulsed by his declaration of love. Despite this, he persevered for a year. The movie Dirty Dancing had just come out, and everyone thought I was a dead ringer for Jennifer Grey. I didn't think I looked like her, but it didn't stop me from trying to dance like her. When I heard Tim was taking another girl to the school dance he instantly became more attractive in my eyes. Before long I fell madly, deeply into my first love.

Tim bore a striking resemblance to David Duchovny from *The X-Files* and never failed to make me laugh. More importantly, he was someone I trusted and whom I could confide in. He looked after me, and was older and more worldly. He soon became my everything. Dad would never have approved of me dating a guy three years my senior. I had no choice but to hide the truth. It didn't take long for my house of lies to tumble. Tim and Anna's mother overheard me on the phone asking my dad if I could sleep at Anna's, even though Anna was going away for the weekend. When I noticed her in the doorway, she was shaking her head disapprovingly.

'Kat Finnerty, I will not stand by while you deceive your poor father. Either you tell him the truth or I will.'

There was no way on God's green earth I was going to tell Dad, so true to her word, she did. Predictably, he hit the roof and forbade the relationship outright, banning me from ever going to their house again, day or night. My refuge was now off-limits. I was ordered to come straight home after school, no clandestine rendezvous. I was beyond devastated. Of course, now I understand Dad's reaction. At 15, I was legally a child; at 18, Tim was not.

Being the headstrong, stubborn soul that I was, within a week of being told the relationship had to end I was sneaking out nearly every night and running to the corner where Tim would be waiting in his parents' idling car. My violin case was tucked into my bed, perfectly shaped as a body double, with an old wig of Mum's resting on the pillow to complete the illusion. Dad had no idea about my night-time escapades but became exasperated by my penchant for challenging virtually every one of his rules. Although none of his boundaries were unreasonable, pushing them was innate to my being. I never took no for an answer.

Of course, being the firstborn meant the rules were far more rigid for me than for my siblings. I felt it was my job to pave the way for them by breaking as many as I could and I took this job very seriously. I was an unguided missile. I skipped classes, had house parties while babysitting, raided the liquor cabinet—but perhaps worst of all, I refused to keep my room tidy. For my father, order was everything, chaos was abhorrent and a messy room was the height of insubordination. He used to shout, 'A messy room is a sign of a messy mind. How can you focus and concentrate on your schoolwork when you're living in a pigsty? CLEAN IT UP!'

Dad grounded me for an entire year after I broke one too many rules. Who gets grounded for a year? Poor Dad, he tried so hard to rein in my wild behaviour. I thought of him as the fun police, and frankly, I felt sorry about his seemingly boring, monotonous life. Work, look after kids, go to church, repeat. The highlight of his day was eating a frozen TV dinner while watching *Coronation Street* on the VCR, which explains why I was so shocked by what happened a few months before my 16th birthday. Out of the blue Dad announced he was marrying Merle, a Guyanese lady who worked with him at the bank. She'd never been married before and had no kids. We'd met her several times, and all of us thought she was okay, except for Martin, who hated her. The night before the wedding I heard him sobbing for what seemed like hours in his room. It broke my heart.

It was a small wedding, and once they were husband and wife, Merle moved in. I wanted Dad to be happy—we all did—so we made a concerted effort to welcome her into our family. But it wasn't long before Merle made it painfully obvious that she was only there to be Dad's wife. She wanted nothing to do with us. Dad now had all of his children to raise, plus a new wife who had no interest in them to keep happy. To his credit, we kids always came first. The pressure must have been hard on him. He had neither the time nor the patience to deal with my ongoing shenanigans. Things finally came to a head one day when I was caught doing the unspeakable.

It was a Saturday night, a few weeks before my 16th birthday. My friend Charmaine was sleeping over, and as a once-off softening of the rules, Dad kindly allowed us to sleep in, which resulted in the missing of 8 a.m. mass. Weekly church attendance was non-negotiable in our house, but by way of compromise, Dad dropped us off at the church for the midday service. We walked in, crossed ourselves with holy water, then walked straight back out, heading for the nearest McDonald's. As we were about to cross the road at the lights, Dad stopped right in front of us. His cigarette nearly fell out of his mouth. I'd never seen him so angry. It would have been more bearable if he'd shouted and screamed, but instead he wordlessly motioned for us to get in the car. The silent treatment continued as we drove home, dropping Charmaine off on the way. I was sick to my stomach with guilt for being caught. I never wanted to disappoint him, but I also felt it was time to stand my ground and tell him the truth. I explained I hated church and didn't believe in God and threw in that he had no right to dictate who I loved.

He regarded me with exasperation, totally at a loss as to what to do with his unruly 15-year-old daughter who'd just renounced God, was fraternising with older boys and still refused to clean her room. Deciding drastic times called for drastic measures, he hauled me to the family GP for some counselling, as one did in those days. Dad walked into the office to lay out the situation. I was left in the waiting room, nervously counting ceiling tiles and biting my nails ragged. Dad finally returned and brusquely grunted, 'Let's go!' Bewildered about how I managed to escape being told off, I sheepishly followed. On the way home, he paraphrased his conversation with the doctor.

'She believes that you're a typical headstrong teenager and that for my own sanity I need to "let go". She told me, "Not every problem is yours to fix." So, my dear daughter, your wish has been granted—you're on your own. I've done all I can. From now on I'm going to let you learn from your own experiences and mistakes. I'm going to "let go and let God".'

He gave me a forlorn glance as he reached for the car cigarette lighter that had just popped.

'Let go and let God?'

Did this mean I could now do what I wanted? No more church? No more curfew? No more groundings? No more boyfriend ban? I'd won! I wanted to do a happy dance. Until I saw the pained look of defeat on my father's face. He didn't say it, but I could almost hear him muttering, 'Why didn't I drown you at birth?'

The joy stemming from the victory of my newfound freedom didn't last long. I began ostracising myself from family and church in an attempt to pursue and justify my own self-interests. But as it turned out, freedom didn't bring me the happiness I thought it would. One afternoon stands out in particular. I'd had a fight with my sister Wendy after she took my answering machine from my room and wouldn't admit to it. So, I kicked down her door and repossessed it. When Dad came home and learnt about the 'karate kid' incident, he berated me for a solid 15 minutes. I felt betrayed. For once little Miss Perfect was in the wrong. She'd stolen from me and lied about it. But I'd been the bad one for so long, I couldn't shake my reputation. Dad hung his head, more deflated than angry, and told me, 'Kat, you know I love you, but I don't like who you are right now.'

The words cut like a knife. My hard-won freedoms turned into a hollow victory. I felt worthless, like I'd let everyone down. I questioned whether I would ever be good enough. After all, Wendy was the best, Martin was the only boy, Caroline and Tracy were sweet little girls who had each other. And then there was me, the black sheep of the family. I looked to my boyfriend for help and support but found none. My euphoric teenage romance had rapidly gone toxic. Tim had slowly turned from a good guy, a friend and a confidant into a drunken, violent control freak. He tried to stop me from spending time with my friends and became dangerously jealous if I did. I found myself isolated from those I was closest to. He told me I was nothing without him. If I argued with him or tried to defy him he'd verbally and physically abuse me. Whenever I tried to break up with him he would cry and tell me how much he loved me, then threaten to hurt me if I ever left him. I was young, naïve and scared. He convinced me that if I lost him, I would never find anyone who would ever love me again.

It was shortly after this that I began to spiral into a deep depression. I was filled with dread and thought my life wasn't worth living. I was selfishly looking at all the things I didn't have rather than being grateful for what I already had. The more I allowed myself to wallow in the perceived emptiness of my life, the more depressed I became. Not even bingeing on brownies and vodka could cure me of my misery. By the time my 16th birthday rolled around I was a mess. Dad tried to cheer me up by presenting me with my mother's favourite bracelet, which he'd been holding on to as a surprise. It was beautiful, a delicate rose gold band, and although I was happy to have a keepsake connecting me to my mother, it was also a grim reminder of everything I'd lost in my life.

Despair crept in, and a sense of worthlessness completely overwhelmed me. It extinguished all the reasons I should have been content with my life. I allowed grief and fear to take over. Destructive thoughts occupied every corner of my mind as I sat alone in my bedroom, hating myself. I made the decision to end my own and everyone else's suffering by jumping off the nearby bridge. I swallowed a handful of aspirin and downed half a bottle of vodka I'd hidden in my underwear drawer. It was exactly 10 p.m. on my 16th birthday when I signed the goodbye note to Dad, opened my window and snuck out for the last time into the cold, dark night.

I walked to the bridge in a trance, focused only on putting an end to my pain. The wind howled and the rain poured, a fitting end to my life and one that mirrored my entry into the world. I wrapped my hands around the thick, icy steel railing and braced myself to climb up and over into the abyss. But as I did so I heard my mother's bracelet chime against the metal. The sound was soothing, like a distant church bell. I thought about my mother and the finality of death, hers and mine. My whole body shook as I wept.

Another death in the family would be devastating for Dad and my siblings. The repercussions and pain would ripple out along with the waves my body would create when I hit the water below. Was it really fair for them to have to wear my pain? Mum had fought so hard to live for all of us and yet, here

I was, thinking about killing myself. Mum didn't have a choice whether she lived or died, but I did. I hesitated, no longer sure I could go through with it. Just then, I heard a car screech to a stop behind me on the bridge.

'Stop, for God's sake, stop!'

It was Dad.

He ran around the car, grabbed me firmly by the scruff of my neck, pulled me back from the railing and shoved me into the front seat of the car. With tears in his eyes, one hand on my shoulder, the other pointing the burning tip of a cigarette at me, he declared fiercely, 'I love you, don't you ever forget that! And if you do anything like that again, you're grounded!'

I looked at my dad and saw deep love, pain and anguish in his eyes. It was as if a veil had suddenly been lifted. And then, before the tears could flow, we started laughing. I'd convinced myself that by taking my life I would be taking away everyone's pain, including my own, but in reality I'd just be transferring my pain to the ones I loved.

Dad was true to his word, I was never grounded again and I learnt a valuable lesson about suffering; in order to avoid transferring my pain to others, I need to be humble enough to reach out for help or courageous enough to confront it. The worst possible action is to internalise and dwell on it. This proved to be fortuitous as I would soon be tested to my physical and mental limits, and this time, the lives of others would depend on how I handled it.

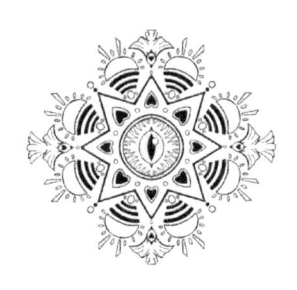

CHAPTER NINE
Toughen Up Buttercup

Strength of character is not always about how much you can handle before you break. It's also about how much you can handle after you've been broken.
~ Robert Tew

The ground was littered with bodies, some writhing and moaning in pain, others motionless. So many casualties. It took a few moments for me to assess the situation and collect my thoughts. I could see the rest of my platoon doing the same. But then our medical training kicked into high gear and we quickly scattered and began triaging. I knelt next to a soldier whose left leg looked to be badly shredded by shrapnel. There was a lot of blood. Maybe the femoral artery had been severed. I knew if I didn't act quickly he would bleed to death, so I dropped to my knees, ripped open some wadding and bandage and applied strong compression to the artery in a bid to stop the bleeding.

My fellow medic tied a tourniquet just above the wound. We then wrapped the bandage tightly around the wadding, rolled the soldier onto a stretcher and elevated his leg as best we could. He was now ready for transport to the field hospital. I looked up at the training assessor for approval, proud I'd remained calm under the intense pressure. He ticked his clipboard.

'Good job Finnerty, now you and Private Johnson get your ass over to the next patient.'

I ran off with a fist pump. I'd come a long way from the emotional, self-absorbed teenager who'd tried to commit suicide two years earlier.

Rewind eight months. I was drunk and stumbling home late at night from a party somewhere in the outer suburbs of Toronto. A taxi pulled to a stop beside me, and I glanced over to see a turban-clad Indian driver with a flowing white beard gesturing for me to climb in. He turned off the meter and offered me a free ride. As I sat in the back, I endured a stern lecture from the big-hearted Sikh, who considered this the price I had to pay for my free passage. At this stage, I'd been living with Charmaine and her family for two years. Dad and I mutually agreed it would be better if I moved out for a while. But just recently he'd finally consented to me moving back home. I was 18 and no longer with Tim. I was single and loving it. My life was one big party.

'Young lady, why are you walking around the streets so late,' admonished the cabbie. 'Nothing good will come of all this drinking and partying. What are you going to do with your life?'

I explained in a slurred voice that I really didn't know what I wanted to do and hadn't really thought too much about it.

He waggled his head, stating, 'You need discipline! You need to join the army.'

Funny how sometimes the most profound wisdom can come from entirely random sources. The next morning, nursing a hangover and feeling a little sad and sorry for myself, I pulled out the phonebook. I'd secretly always harboured a dream to enlist in the Peace Corps and took the wise cabbie's pronouncement as a sign. Unfortunately, the Peace Corps wasn't in the white or yellow pages. Hell, I wasn't even sure they existed in Canada. I looked up the armed forces as an alternative. Sailing around the world on a ship with the navy also sounded like a blast. The recruiters immediately made an appointment for me to come in for an interview. Basic training was about to begin for the reserves.

Two weeks later, Dad proudly dropped me off at the downtown barracks. I was taken north by bus into the middle of Ontario where there was a distinct lack of ocean. On arrival, I was handed some green fatigues, which was confusing.

'Where are the boats and the blue uniforms?' I asked the corporal.

'You joined the army, you idiot, not the navy. There are no boats.'

Visions of the hell Private Benjamin experienced flashed through my mind. Army, Navy, it was all the same. And if it was anything like Goldie's experience, I was going to love it! After all, the army were experts at building strength from pain, and this rather appealed to my warped, slightly masochistic nature. As expected, the physical training was brutal, but contrary to most sane people, it was my idea of bliss. It's not that I enjoyed the pain—well, maybe I did just a little—but rather that I got off on the endorphin hit and the challenge and the fact I was burning calories. It meant I could eat more cake and drink more beer without the side effect of a fat gut! Sadly, cake and beer were noticeably absent in the mess hall during basic training.

Part of our army conditioning involved being kept awake for five days to prepare us for real warfare. We'd be so tired during these training exercises that when we were given the command to stand down, everyone would simply drop and fall asleep where they were standing, even if it was in a pile of prickly pine needles. Our rest would last no more than five minutes before we'd be ordered to march on. I kept reminding myself of the Japanese proverb, 'Fall down seven times, get up eight'. It's amazing what your mind and body can tolerate when pushed to the edge. We all have limits, but the army taught me that most of our limits are self-imposed. We can push past them if we have to. Many nights were spent in muddy trenches looking for non-existent enemies. The only real threat was from the forest. It was full of bears. The division was on a budget, so instead of blanks in our semi-automatic rifles, we had to say 'bang-bang' in a loud voice. We hoped the bears knew how to play dead.

Most of the platoon leaders were tough, but Sergeant Schneider was by far the worst. He was particularly cruel to me, and I often suffered at his hands. 'Why is he always picking on me?' I would wonder to myself. At this stage in my life I had no concept of karma, otherwise I would have reflected back on all the times I'd been similarly brutal to my siblings. Sergeant Schneider would get in my face and shower me with saliva while barking orders. If I made any indication of wiping my face, he'd punish the platoon and sneer, 'Toughen up Buttercup.' The harder he pushed me, the more determined I was to hold my ground. He tried his best to break me, but I refused to remain broken. To this day, I still use my darkest hours of pain and most difficult situations as catalysts for change, for growth, for building resilience. They are the times I look in the mirror, see the eyes of my enemy staring back at me and say, 'Time to toughen up Buttercup!'

The army taught us we were neither male nor female, simply soldiers. We were no longer individuals but part of a well-honed team. We were only ever as good as the weakest person in the platoon. We survived by helping one another, and lived and breathed the motto 'we before me'. Such camaraderie was something I'd never experienced before and haven't felt since. It was eye-opening and enlightening and taught me the value of being a team player and the true meaning of discipline.

I now understood why Dad had imposed so many rules at home. He wasn't the fun police; he was simply trying to keep us safe, organised and in line. If there was no discipline, no God or King to answer to, we'd have done whatever we wanted without considering the needs, wants and well-being of others or the ramifications of our actions. Poor Dad—the needless hell I'd put him through.

With six weeks of basic training completed, we graduated and commenced our advanced training to become medics. It was intense but oh so much fun! We were, in essence, a MASH unit, part of a mobile army surgical hospital. Just like on the TV show, there was joy and pain and the occasional shedding of tears—others, not mine of course. We spent hours learning how to deal with major trauma injuries resulting from explosions and gunshots. We learnt to improvise splints and stretchers from the bush around us, and I discovered it was possible to lift someone much heavier than myself in an over-the-shoulder 'fireman carry'. This helped immensely on those nights when some of us drank too much and couldn't walk home.

Towards the end of my stint in the army, there was one incident I'll never forget. I hatched a plan to go drinking at a nearby bar, but that meant having to go AWOL, a highly punishable offence. To pull it off I needed someone on the inside, someone I could trust. So I enlisted the help of none other than my arch-enemy, Sergeant Schneider. Turned out that when he was not playing the asshole drill sergeant in basic training, he was actually an okay kinda guy. He was also my occasional drinking buddy.

Under the cover of darkness I climbed into the boot of his car. The last thing I saw and heard as the boot slammed shut was Sergeant Schneider grinning maniacally and saying, 'Time to toughen up Buttercup!' Suffice to say, we made it undetected through the sentry post, although he did make me sweat it out for quite a few more kilometres than necessary before he pulled over. We spent the next few hours bonding over pints and pool, and I successfully made it back to camp undetected.

As a result of these and other incidents, I came to realise that sometimes your worst enemy, your harshest critic, turns out to be your best teacher. I now try to regularly step outside my comfort zone and celebrate every little victory as one more way to grow strong and overcome the Sergeant Schneiders of the world. The old adage is true, what doesn't kill you makes you stronger as long as you understand that there's always a lesson hidden within the struggle, and you make the effort to find it.

Not long after this, my regiment of reserve medics was deemed redundant and disbanded. Our job was to save lives, but seeing as Canada wasn't actively involved in any wars at the time, there were no lives to save. I left with an honourable discharge, which impressed Father to no end. He was certain I would go AWOL. And I *had* gone AWOL of course—I just didn't get caught! I returned home with a new attitude and a great deal more respect for Dad's rules. Then I screwed it all up by joining a cult.

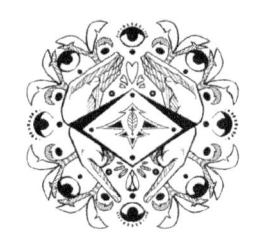

CHAPTER TEN
The Cult of Personality

People who fail focus on what they have to go through; people who succeed focus on what it will feel like at the end.
~ Tony Robbins

My indoctrination into the cult began innocuously enough. I was outside my local 7-Eleven, juggling a bagful of Twizzlers, my favourite candy, when a long-haired, middle-aged man in a cheap suit approached me. It was a typical Toronto summer's day; hot, dry and windy. I was 19, fresh out of the army, and living back at Dad's place. *Jumping Jehoshaphat,* I thought. *What the hell does this guy want?*

I attempted to unlock my car door and make a speedy getaway, all while trying to hold down my wind-blown miniskirt and shove a Twizzler into my mouth, but I'd barely grasped the door handle when he materialised next to me.

'Hey there,' he smiled as he thrust his hand towards me. 'My name is Glenn. Do you like to eat?'

And that was how I met my first coupon cult member. Glenn proceeded to tell me about a two-for-one coupon I couldn't live without. I tried to excuse myself, but he was very persuasive. When I realised the coupons were for meals at my favourite pub, I happily handed over 20 bucks. Bargain. As I made to slide into my car, he placed a gentle hand on my arm.

'Look, I don't normally hang out in parking lots. I was picking up my suits at the dry cleaner when I saw you. I like to think of myself as a good judge of character, and I can tell by chatting with you that you're the type who seizes an opportunity when presented with one.'

I sighed, offering him a Twizzler. He had me pegged. I was a sucker for anything new or adventurous.

Glenn flashed a yellow-toothed grin.

'Just give me five minutes of your time. Have I got an opportunity for you!'

I rolled my eyes.

He pulled a wad of cash from his inside pocket.

'No, really. There's huge money in this marketing business. You're friendly, outgoing, cute—you'd be perfect for the job.' He moved closer, lowering his voice. 'Of course, you'll need to get through a strict interview process, but I'd love to have you on my team. I can put in a good word.'

Everything screamed scam, but what can I say? I was curious, unemployed and bored. Glenn gave me the address of the company's office, and before I knew it I was on my way to a warehouse in the industrial part of town to meet the company director, a smartly dressed Italian in an Armani suit accessorised with flashy jewellery. He had perfectly styled hair, mesmerising eyes, and a voice so smooth it dripped honey and left me hanging on his every word. His name was Tony Bacardi. By the time I left his office he'd convinced me I'd soon be flying around the world first class if I was accepted for the job. And just like anyone else who could fog a mirror, I got the gig.

The next day, I arrived at 8 a.m. sharp, dressed as instructed, in business attire with comfortable walking shoes. I was excited about my new adventure. Glenn beamed when he saw me and congratulated me on being brought on board. He then introduced me to his three-man team, all of whom looked as though they'd been recruited from the local methadone clinic. A gong sounded, and about 50 of us, mostly men, piled into a windowless room covered with inspirational posters and motivational quotes. The lights dimmed, and music began to play. Everyone was eerily still and silent. It was creepy, but I was intrigued to see what would happen next. A door opened, and a smiling Tony sauntered in with all the coolness of Fonzie. The group went wild, clapping, chanting and reaching out to touch him. Looking around, I wondered if they'd been drinking from the same pitcher of Kool-Aid. Tony gave out high fives as he made his way around the room. When he reached me he stopped, flashed me his million-dollar smile, winked and held up his bejewelled hand. I high-fived him back. Stuff it, I was all in.

For the next hour, we sat on the floor, transfixed, as Tony preached a never-ending stream of motivational clichés.

'Every day is the beginning of the rest of your life.'

'The decisions you make right now will shape your destiny.'

'Every moment of every day, you decide who you are and what you believe in.'

'There is no past, only future. Every second you get a second chance.'

His words were hypnotic; they pushed all my buttons, and he was a consummate showman.

'You have a chance now to take on this amazing opportunity, but you have to work for it. All of you here are special because you've chosen to change your life. You will make a difference in the world, not just by saving people money with coupons but also by making so much money you will transform your life.'

I noted the expectant faces surrounding me.

'Imagine being able to take your families and friends on exotic holidays. Dedicate yourself to the company, be a team player, work hard for a few years following our system. This is your path to success.'

'The System', I would later learn, involved building up a team of salespeople who in turn would recruit their own team. You received a percentage of every sale made by everyone on your team. It was a classic pyramid scheme designed to make those at the top filthy rich. I was young and naïve, unaware of the ramifications. At the end of the sermon we all went mad, clapping and chanting, 'Every no leads to a yes! Every no leads to a yes!' We marched outside, super-pumped, ready to sell. It was pouring rain. We pulled up to our first underground parking lot. Turns out Glenn was pretty familiar with parking lots.

On my very first day I smashed it, selling 25 coupons—a record for a newbie. I hit the gong three times when we returned, soaking wet, later that night. Everyone congratulated me as if I'd just won Olympic gold.

I loved my new job. I was walking all day—not stuck behind a desk—meeting people, chatting, being social and learning the fine art of cold calling. The number one rule was that before people buy what you're selling, they have to buy into you; your personality, your smile, your ability to empathise and listen. Getting strangers from all walks of life to like and trust you enough to hand over twenty bucks to buy a coupon isn't easy, but I always considered it a personal challenge. Besides, compared to an irate drill sergeant yelling abuse at me, this was a walk in the park. I told myself that every door slammed in my face would get me closer to the one that opens and that if a door didn't open, it was because it was never meant to. I learned not to take rejection personally, that it was a just numbers game, a means to an end, the goal being to become a wildly successful coupon mogul.

In my spare time, I devoured the motivational books Tony lent me. It proved to be one of the many turning points in my life. My mind was awakened to the world of self-help gurus. I learnt how to view every crappy situation as an opportunity for growth and learning. My favourite book was Anthony Robbins' *Awaken the Giant Within*. 'Every adversity in life has the seed of an equal or greater benefit hidden within it' became my mantra. I now knew exactly where I wanted to end up, and it wasn't selling coupons in parking lots. I had awakened the giant within, and there was no stopping me.

I moved into my first apartment and, within a short time, had the biggest sales team at the office. I was consistently the highest seller and received large weekly bonuses. Money started rolling in from my team. Visions of lounging by an infinity pool, sipping daiquiris while gazing at the pool boy over my sunnies began to seem like an achievable reality. I was 20 years old and managing a crew of ten guys, some of whom were much older and better educated than I was. I utilised everything I'd learnt so far in my life in order to keep my team inspired and driven. I was on top of the world. My future was golden. Until, less than six months later, everything came to an unexpectedly frosty end.

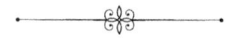

One chilly autumn morning, after yet another of Tony's inspirational meetings, he called me into his office to introduce me to an up-and-coming manager from another district. He was a few years older than me and had an athletic build with preppy, pretty-boy good looks. He oozed charisma. No wonder he was so high up in the company, I thought. He shook my hand, holding my gaze confidently as he introduced himself.

'Hi gorgeous, name's Gord, like God with an R,' he chuckled. 'It's wonderful to finally meet you. Been hearing a lot about you and your team.'

Butterflies erupted in my belly. I was struck down by a full-blown schoolgirl crush. Tony had chosen Gord to open up western Canada and, apparently, they needed someone like me to join the team. Would I be interested? If there's one thing I truly despise, it's the cold—a bold statement coming from a born-and-bred Canadian. The idea of freezing my butt off selling coupons door to door in one of the country's coldest climates didn't exactly appeal to me. All I can say in my defence is that love can lead you to the strangest of places.

Three days later I found myself squeezed into Gord's beat-up Toyota, along with two other top coupon salesmen, ready to make the 3,000 km drive west. It was a long, cold journey, but by the time we arrived at the frozen city of Saskatoon, Saskatchewan, Gord and I were firmly in love, or lust—not sure quite which. Had Gord not convinced me of his undying affection and commitment, had I not been completely sold on his promises, I doubt I would have stayed more than a few days in the city.

It was January, and the region was experiencing one of their worst winters on record: blizzards, white-outs and days when the temperature plunged to -60°C. Exposed skin froze in minutes. It was horrendous, definitely not favourable working conditions for a door-to-door salesperson. People wouldn't even open their doors for fear of letting the heat out and cold in. Walking those streets was sheer madness, yet there we were, nearly dying from exposure for the dream we'd been sold.

Gord, being the boss, sat in a toasty warm office all day with a personal secretary making him coffee. Sales were terrible, and he blamed me. We started arguing. He felt I wasn't doing enough to sign up new recruits. I thought he should get his ass off his warm leather chair and spend a day outside with us. I began questioning my decision to leave behind my successful team in Toronto.

One bitterly cold day the ice beneath my new reality finally cracked. I was working with a fresh recruit, knocking doors on the outskirts of town, when a man opened the door, looked me over and invited me in. I didn't even give it a second thought, I was so relieved to get out of the cold. He seemed friendly at first, but things quickly turned nasty. He grabbed my arm and tried to shut the door behind me. I screamed for help, but the new recruit didn't hear me as he was on the other side of the road. Luckily, I was wearing about 12 layers of clothing. My puffy, damp jacket slipped through the man's hands, giving me time to stumble back out the door. I sprinted as fast as I could across the road and explained to the recruit in heaving breaths what just happened. He was shocked and asked what I wanted to do.

'I'm done. I'm finished. We are outta here,' I stated emphatically, even though we weren't due back at the office for another three hours. All I could think of was falling into Gord's safe, strong arms.

By the time I reached the office I was wet, dirty, cold, and angry. I marched past the front desk on which sat a copy of the local newspaper. The front page featured Gord's picture and a headline that screamed, *Coupon Company a Cult!* I pushed open his door, and that's when I realised Sasha the secretary wasn't sitting in her usual chair. She was straddling Gord's. A fresh cup of steaming coffee was teetering precariously on his desk. I was floored. The only thing I could think of to say was, 'Oh God, I mean…Gord, I should have knocked.' I turned and slammed the door and left. And suddenly, it was as though I'd broken through the ice. My vision cleared. Scenes from the past 18 months flashed before my eyes, like I was an actress in a B-grade rom-com gone wrong. I realised my relationship was over, along with my love of coffee and my stellar career as a door-to-door salesperson.

The next morning I boarded a plane back to Toronto. Sadly, the dreams of a luxury mansion complete with sexy pool guy never eventuated, but honestly, in my heart of hearts I didn't really care. When I landed in Toronto and the sun lit up the wet runway like a magical silver rainbow, I had a revelation. Although I was in a crappy situation, I could see there was a seed of equal or greater benefit wrapped within it. Italian Stallion Tony, Anthony Robbins and the cult had opened my eyes to a whole new world, one filled with self-help books, motivational seminars, advanced sales techniques and personal development. My cult experience wasn't a write-off; it had equipped me with the ability to use my thoughts to shape my destiny. I decided that as soon as I made it home I would put my newfound powers of manifestation to the test. And amazingly, they worked! I just never expected my dreams to manifest so quickly or in quite such a bizarre manner.

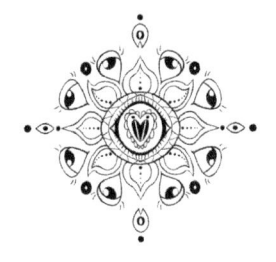

CHAPTER ELEVEN
The Bachelor Auction

Nothing lasts forever so live it up;
drink it down, laugh it off, avoid the drama,
Take chances and never have regrets because,
at one point, everything you did was exactly what you wanted.
~ Marilyn Monroe

Escaping the company cult and breaking up with God with an R proved to be a Godsend. Within weeks I'd found my new calling: selling memberships for a high-end gym in Toronto. I now had a warm office and a secretary. Shame I was still off coffee. In my new job I was able to apply the techniques I'd learnt in my door-knocking days, but because I was already passionate about fitness, it meant I could put my heart and soul into the sales. I made good money and, as a bonus, I pumped some serious iron with my co-workers.

We were a tight-knit bunch of muscle-bound friends who ate way too many egg whites and spent far too much time looking at ourselves in mirrors. I was soon the fittest I'd ever been—I finally achieved a six-pack! Life was great. The more thankful I became, the more content I was and the better my life seemed to flow. Then member #301 entered my life. His name was Hugh, and he was hot. Aunt Kath would have called him 'a dish'. Every day at 5:30 p.m. he arrived wearing a tailor-made suit, tie draped around his neck, a few shirt buttons undone. Hugh was tall, well-built, with short, dark wavy hair and striking blue-green eyes. Just knowing he was in the same building made my stomach flip. I'd lurk at the front desk just to catch a glimpse of him but never actually spoke to him. Oh no, no way. I was petrified of having a conversation, content to discreetly admire him from behind the safety of the desk while my imagination ran wild.

One of my co-workers was a divinely gorgeous Aussie guy named Clark. We were great friends. One day in late October he invited the receptionist Jenn and I to an exclusive gala being held to raise funds for the Multiple Sclerosis Society. There was to be a bachelor auction, and Clark was one of the 20 men up for bids. Apart from being sexy and single, participants were also required to find sponsors who would donate holidays, airfares, dinners at fancy restaurants, or any other upmarket prize that could be finagled. The highest bidder won a combo package: the goods and the guy on a holiday for two.

It was a high-class extravaganza at the Toronto Convention Centre. At $250 a ticket, it wasn't the type of lavish event I would normally fork out for, but Jenn and I decided we'd splurge so we could support Clark's philanthropic endeavour of donating himself to a worthy cause. We bought gowns that Cinderella would have envied, had our hair done and bits of our bodies waxed. We looked the part, even if we felt more comfortable in sneakers than stilettos. When we arrived, we were given gold-embossed booklets with the line-up of bachelors. Clark's profile was there, but to my utter astonishment, so was Hugh's! I couldn't believe that in a city of 10 million, the guy of my daydreams was one of the 20 eligible bachelors. And bingo, now I knew he was single. I needed a drink!

We mingled with the rich and richer of Toronto's elite, sipping flutes of expensive champagne. Truth be told, I had the waiter top up my glass more than a few times. There were hundreds of people dressed in ball gowns and black ties, all looking distinguished and glamorous. Then there was me, gym membership chick at The Workout. I still had the price tags of my dress tucked in at the back so I could return it the next day. I felt like an imposter.

An attractive middle-aged woman in a wheelchair took to the stage to kick off the event. She shared her experiences of living with multiple sclerosis. Her speech was slurred, and it was an effort to understand her, but I found myself listening intently to every word. It was a tragic story.

'I was on my honeymoon when I started seeing black spots in my right eye. I'd just turned 25, and my husband and I were looking forward to filling our house with children,' she said. 'At the time I was working as a midwife, and it wasn't long before I fell pregnant with our daughter. After she was born, my health deteriorated rapidly and I was diagnosed with primary progressive MS. Months later my legs became so weak I needed a walker.'

She looked around and took a shaky breath. The audience was silent, both out of respect for her courage and because, like me, they were caught up in her story.

'The worst was when I lost control over my bladder. My husband is a doctor, so we tried anything and everything to cure me. We spared no expense. However, it wasn't long before I was unable to look after myself, let alone my child.'

As she gazed out over the attendees, her eyes seemed to land on mine. For the briefest of moments, I felt we connected.

'I knew it was going to be easier for my family if I was cared for in a nursing home. And that was probably the hardest decision of all.'

I looked down at my ball gown and designer shoes, ashamed that only moments earlier I'd been obsessing over whether I measured up to my fellow guests, whether I looked glamorous enough—petty thoughts compared to what this woman was going through every day of her life. I glanced back up as she added, 'But it's not so bad. My husband and daughter visit most weekends, and on special occasions we go somewhere nice for dinner.'

The room was silent. How could she stand being a prisoner in a body that no longer functioned? I couldn't begin to imagine what her life was like. I closed my eyes and tried to concentrate on her words.

'I'm 45, but I live the life of a 90-year-old. MS doesn't usually kill you; you just suffer one debilitating attack after another, each one leaving you more disabled than before. Treatments are mostly ineffective. There's no cure.'

My heart broke imagining her pain, and I felt a palpable, almost guilty relief when the speech ended and the bachelor auction began. I think we all did. The first of many sharply dressed men began strutting across the stage. They boasted extravagant prize packages: safaris in Africa, shopping sprees in Paris, a wine tour through the Chianti region of Italy. As a result, several bachelors incited bidding wars that ended up well over ten grand. The rich old gals were spending up big. I was relieved for Clark when his winning bidder was a nice-looking blonde.

Then came my gym guy. Hugh's trip wasn't anywhere near as exciting as the others—a four-day getaway to Florida—but at least the accommodation was five-star. Bidding kicked off low and slow. I felt bad for him striding up and down the stage as the auctioneer attempted to convince the crowd he was worth more than $4,000. With champagne-soaked judgement, I found my hand shooting up of its own volition.

'Five thousand,' I yelled confidently. Jenn stared at me in disbelief and slapped her forehead.

'Five grand? Are you completely crazy?'

'Jenny, the way I see it, if no one's ever called you crazy, you're just not doing life right. Besides, it's not as if I'm going to win. I'm just helping the guy out.'

She peered at me, eyebrows raised. I smiled and toasted her with another full glass of champers. Just then we heard the auctioneer call out, 'Going once to the lady at table 20.'

Dead silence.

'Going twice.'

'Please tell me this isn't happening,' I groaned to myself.

'Going three times...sold to the lucky lass at the back of the room. Come on up and meet your bachelor.'

Time stood still. Oh no! Did I just buy Gym Guy? My first thoughts were, why didn't someone outbid me? And wait, what did I just blow five grand on, apart from Hugh? I glanced down at the booklet, and there it was: a few days in Miami, a couple of dinners at an Italian restaurant, a year of free tanning, and a week's supply of designer underwear. Damn, if only I hadn't had that last glass of bubbly. I'd just donated the deposit on my new car.

I felt a tap on my shoulder as one of the bidding spotters handed me a rose to present to Hugh. I stood up and began to walk from the back of the massive ballroom to the front. All eyes were on me. In my mind, I glided elegantly through the crowd, across the dance floor and up the steps towards the man of my dreams. In reality, I was in a champagne-addled state, tottering and swaying in heels that were far too high for me. At some point I think I knocked over an empty chair. When I finally arrived at the stairs there was a moment of panic—I desperately hoped the price tags weren't hanging out of the back of my dress.

I held the auctioneer's hand as he guided me across the stage. Hugh looked profoundly befuddled.

'Aren't you the chick that works at my gym?'

'Umm...yes,' I mumbled.

My hand trembled as I gave him the flower. I barely had the courage to look him in the eyes.

Spending five grand on Hugh was about as subtle a pick-up as a lap dance. As we linked arms and stepped off stage, immediate payment was requested. Thankfully I had an American Express card hidden in the glove box of my car. As I'd promised the telemarketer who convinced me to apply for it, I never left home without it. It was 1995, and credit cards with smart chips were just becoming popular in Europe and America, along with personal mobile phones and the mass adoption of something called the world wide web. Hugh kindly offered to accompany me to my car. I was still in shock over what had just happened. I stared at the ground, scared I might trip, too nervous to make eye contact. As we waited for the elevator, I cleared my throat and attempted to clarify.

'I didn't mean to buy you. I was just trying to help. I didn't think you'd go so cheap.'

Oh my God, I couldn't believe I'd just said that. I wanted to curl up and disappear.

Hugh laughed with good humour.

'Thanks...I think.'

Then we were alone in the elevator, and the muzak descended on us, a classic keyboard version of 'You Make Me Feel Like A Natural Woman'. Yet another layer of awkwardness. I looked intently at the numbers, studiously avoiding Hugh's gaze. The music wasn't nearly loud enough to drown out the sound of my pounding heart. I felt him move closer, then there he was, right in front of me. He pulled me firmly but gently towards him. I felt light-headed and thought I might pass out. I couldn't believe this was happening. I'd imagined this scene a million times in my mind. I'd even memorised his member profile. Hell, I knew his mother's name, Glenice, and that she was his emergency contact. Hugh didn't even know my name.

My chest heaved under my padded push-up bra. I could feel his perfectly chiselled muscles through his tuxedo. My body shuddered with desire. I was slightly queasy—the champagne might well have been a contributing factor—my eyes were squeezed shut.

'Open your eyes.'

I looked up, nearly drowning in his intoxicating blue-green gaze

In a husky voice, he murmured, 'I'm so glad it was you who bought me...Kat.'

I gasped. He knew my name? Before I could react he leaned down, held my face in his hands and gently kissed me.

'And Kat,' he whispered.

'Mmmm,' I said dreamily.

'Just so you know, you didn't have to buy me... I would have been yours for free.'

I groaned in exasperation, banging my head back against the elevator wall. Bloody liquid courage just cost me five grand! When would I ever learn? But by the time the elevator door opened at P5, he was kissing me again and I figured, what the hell, it's worth the ride. My daydream had manifested itself.

The next few weeks were a blur as Hugh and I fell into a passionate relationship. However, by the time we arrived in Miami four months later for our official package holiday, my shudders of desire and the burning inferno of my initial passion had dwindled down to a flickering candle flame. Things hadn't quite turned out the way I'd hoped. I wasn't too upset. Here I was staying at a five-star hotel, dining at Miami's finest restaurants and, even though Hugh and I weren't in love, he made for great eye candy. But the whole time I was away I couldn't shake the image of the lady from the bachelor auction sitting in her wheelchair in the nursing home, eating puréed food and waiting for her weekly family visit. Compared with losing a man I'd lusted after for a year and spent five grand on, I had nothing to complain about.

And that's the thing about perspective. In order to maintain it, you have to consistently perform some brutally honest comparison shopping and regularly ask yourself, 'Are my problems really that bad or do I just think they are?' Most of us who live in the first world are scab pickers. We obsess about the little problems and pick at them until they bleed. Worse, we often blow these problems way out of proportion thanks to our skewed sense of self-importance.

It took the lady at the bachelor auction to put everything into perspective for me. Time to stop complaining about what I didn't have and start being grateful for what I did have, beginning with my health. Because, deep down, I knew I'd rather be dead than living with MS.

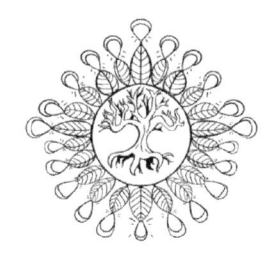

CHAPTER TWELVE
Feel the Fear and Do It Anyway

If you knew you could handle everything that came your way, what would you possibly have to fear? The answer is: nothing!
~ Susan Jeffers

Prior to my psychic reading, I was an overly confident 23-year-old leading an ordinary life in Toronto, working, partying with friends and generally feeling pretty good about myself. However, within months of the reading, I found myself winging my way to the other side of the world in search of the meaning of life on the 'Island of the Gods'. This spontaneous quest for adventure would take me within a whisker of dying and leave me scarred for life.

How did this happen? Let's start with the psychic. It's not like I was a devout Ouija board-carrying follower of all things mystical. I was a street-savvy sceptic, thanks in part to my brief coupon cult experience. But for some reason, I felt drawn to the elderly woman in the shopping mall that day. Perhaps it had something to do with her compassionate eyes, or that she didn't look like a whack job but more like an elderly, well-dressed grandmother, sitting quietly in her tiny kiosk. This was comforting given it wasn't exactly normal for a psychic to be set up next to my favourite coffee shop.

I found myself squeezing into the chair opposite her. She smiled and said knowingly, 'I'm glad you chose to see me, dear. There's something important I need to tell you about your future.'

My heart skipped a beat. Please don't tell me I'm about to die.

The last psychic I'd seen was over ten years ago when Mum felt the urge to visit one while on our annual holiday at Wasaga Beach. Mum was the picture of good health at the time, running around after five kids. There were no signs she would be dead within a year, but during the reading she was told she'd become gravely ill. The psychic was so concerned she'd given Mum the contact details for a healer, the same one we drove 1,400 km to visit several months later. I remember that Hail Mary run clear as day, a last-ditch attempt to save her. Despite all the effort, she'd died anyway. Fate? Destiny? Could Mum have changed the outcome if she'd seen the healer or the doctors sooner? It was impossible to speculate. As I sat opposite my own clairvoyant, I began wondering what exactly I was in for.

She took my hand in hers, closed her eyes and began describing the kids I swore I was never going to have, two boys and a girl, blonde hair, blue eyes. I laughed at the unimaginable. Here we go, I thought.

'I feel there's an emptiness inside you at the moment,' she continued, 'a void that won't be filled here in Canada. I'm sensing you're destined to help people, but first you'll go through some painful times.'

Okay lady, so far I think I've just wasted 20 bucks.

'You need to leave here and travel overseas to find out who you really are.'

My scepticism was kicking into high gear. Kind of a no-brainer given that most young people have a desire to travel and 'find' themselves. Then she stopped mid-sentence, opened her eyes and stared at me with an intensity that freaked me out.

'Your leg, your left leg, there's something wrong with it. You're struggling to put on your shoe.'

I couldn't help but laugh. I'd been bracing myself for something much worse.

'Well, the only leg problem I have is that my quads are killing me from the workout I did yesterday. So yes, I did struggle to put my shoes on this morning.'

She looked confused. This was obviously not the response she was looking for.

In the end, I was relieved my destiny involved travel and helping people rather than illness and imminent death. I was still a little unsure of the psychic's accuracy, though she was right about one thing: I did have a growing hole in my soul. I was desperate for more adventure, meaning and purpose in my life. Yes, I was having fun but I didn't feel content. Life in

Toronto was one party after another, and my biggest concern revolved around how many hours of cardio I needed to do to keep my 'muffin top' from protruding over the waistband of my leggings. My hedonistic lifestyle—hanging with friends at trendy pubs and clubs and working on my figure and bank balance—wasn't exactly delivering me a life full of meaning and satisfaction.

As I walked through the mall, the words on a book cover in a store window caught my eye: *Feel the Fear and Do It Anyway!* I was a sucker for a good self-help book, and those seven words called out to me. I took it home and read it over dinner, devouring the chapters as voraciously as my egg white omelette. Susan Jeffers' insights resonated with my innermost thoughts.

'Pushing through fear is less frightening than living with the bigger underlying fear that comes from a feeling of helplessness! When you push through the fear, you will feel such a sense of relief as your feeling of helplessness subsides. You will wonder why you did not take action sooner.'

Here I was, a little bored and lost, wanting more out of my life, living with the fear of leaving my cushy job, friends and comfortable lifestyle. I was a walking contradiction! Susan Jeffers was right. It was time to act, time to 'feel the fear and do it anyway'. But where to go and what to do? I had a flashback to when I was a little girl, lying on my top bunk, staring out the window at the icicles hanging from the eaves. I'd shine my flashlight on the shards of ice, imagining the reflected light as that of a blistering Australian sun. I was infatuated with the idea of a land down under. A land as sunny and hot as mine was cold and dark, a land full of koalas and kangaroos and bronzed Aussies with cool accents, like Sandy from *Grease*. Australia...why not? It was the ultimate travel adventure destination and the perfect place to challenge myself. But first I had to convince my bestie to come with me. I wasn't quite ready to face my fears alone.

As it turned out, Layla didn't need much convincing. She was all in the moment I mentioned Australia. Layla was a stunner: tall, blonde, perfect body, a Playboy centrefold, the trophy wife most men desired. Hanging out with her was great. I called her 'Man Burley' for her ability to attract the best-looking fish. Her relationships and engagements never lasted long, and I was often the beneficiary of diamond rings originally destined for her perfect fingers. I forged ahead with my travel plans. The cheapest flights I could find to Australia were with Garuda, an airline I'd never heard of, via an island I didn't even know existed: Bali. I looked it up in a Lonely Planet guide. 'The Island of the Gods. A Tropical Paradise'. It sounded perfect! Days before our departure, Layla rocked me with the news she wouldn't be coming. She was in love, and this time she was sure he was the one.

Layla's pull-out at the 11th hour sent me into a tailspin, and my biggest fear—loneliness—reared its ugly head. I hated the idea of being alone, partly because I was social by nature and partly because it meant I didn't have to think about life's deeper questions.

Once the disappointment subsided, I thought, *No excuses. If I can create my own suffering, I can also create my own joy. All I need to do is adopt a different mindset and become a braver version of myself.* Here was an opportunity to do something I'd dreamt about since I was a child, maybe even a chance to 'fill the hole in my soul' and find more meaning and purpose in my life. What did Susan Jeffers say?

'Commit to the fear and push through it to become more than you are now in the present.'

Suddenly I knew, with absolute conviction, that if I wanted to embrace change and growth, I'd have to put my fear of loneliness aside and go it alone. Not surprisingly, my propensity for sniffing out trouble meant my attempts to fill the hole in my soul actually ended up with me tearing a hole in my body instead.

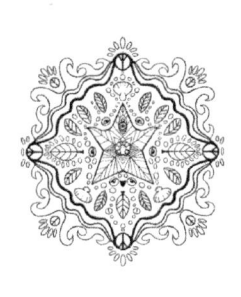

CHAPTER THIRTEEN
Island of the Gods

All the suffering in the world comes from thinking of oneself.
All the happiness in the world comes from thinking of others.
- Shantideva

If first impressions are everything, then the start of my epic journey to Australia via Bali didn't bode well. The Garuda plane, part of the official airline fleet of Indonesia, was old and reeked of smoke—yes, you could still smoke on some airlines in the 90s—and I found myself spending the next 15 hours breathing in a hazy cloud of toxic cigarette fumes. By the time we landed in Bali, I had a raging headache and a sore throat, which intensified when I discovered the main tourist town of Kuta was not the calm, tropical oasis I'd read about, but a chaotic, noisy, smelly metropolis.

Island of the Gods? Seriously? Manic motorbike riders zipped around the streets in their hundreds, barely missing any pedestrians brave enough to attempt to cross. Cars and buses competed to out-honk each other, accompanied by yelling street hawkers and roadside bars cranking out thumping baselines. It was crazy, miles from my idea of paradise. A beat-up taxi drove me past the high-walled beachside resorts of the rich and into the back streets of Kuta. It was dark when we pulled up to an open-air pub filled with drunken Aussie tourists singing 'I come from a land down under'. A man at a food cart was selling chicken satay cooked over hot coals. A skinny woman lay curled next to him on a mat on the dirty sidewalk, a baby cradled in her arms.

I staggered down a dark, narrow alley, my backpack and growing worries weighing me down until I arrived at a quaint, ornate building called Wayan's Homestay. I sighed with relief. My $5-a-night accommodation didn't look too bad. A small, round-faced Balinese man introduced himself as Wayan. His front desk was adorned with an eclectic mix of religious offerings, wooden carvings, fresh flowers, and a plastic ornamental cat with rocking arms. He walked me to my room along an intricately laid pebble path surrounded by lush gardens. I pushed open a flimsy bamboo door to reveal a clean but spartan room with a single bed. After thanking him, I closed the door and collapsed on the thin mattress, trying my best to hold back the tsunami of tears that threatened to engulf me as the reality of my loneliness hit me. It seemed the hole in my soul had followed me. I was still suffering, except now the suffering was framed by palm trees and the thin bamboo walls of Wayan's Homestay in Paradise.

Sleep was a next-to-impossible task given the mixture of jet lag, buzzing mosquitoes, barking dogs and roosters crowing long before first light. As soon as the sun came up I decided to make the best of it and do what made me happy: run! I found my way to the beach and jogged until my belly growled. I arrived back at Wayan's on a sweaty endorphin high. Entering the tiny eating area, I noticed a good-looking older guy with shaggy blond hair and smiling blue eyes devouring a giant pancake. Things were looking up already.

'I'll have what he's having,' I called out hungrily to Wayan.

The blond man laughed and gestured for me to join him at his table.

'Name's Ash.'

'I'm Kat.'

I tried to wipe my hand dry before shaking his, only partially achieving success.

'Sorry, sweaty hands, just been for a run.'

I couldn't help but notice he looked a lot like an older version of Matthew McConaughey. His accent was from the American South, a honeyed southern drawl.

'Well now, what in the Sam Hill would possess you to run around in this here sauna?'

'Running makes me happy.'

'As good an answer as any,' he grinned. 'So whatcha y'all doin' here?'

'No y'all.' I shrugged. 'Just me. Got in last night. To be honest I'm not sure why I'm here.'

He widened his eyes in amused curiosity, so I elaborated.

'Bali is just a stopover. I'm on my way to Australia. What about you?'

Ash explained he'd spent the last few years travelling through Asia, sourcing unique, handcrafted jewellery from local villages and communities for his business.

'My real passion is philanthropy and the philosophy of fair trade. You know, giving people a hand up rather than a handout. I run a business with a mission of purpose.'

The jewellery he collected was in high demand back in the US because each piece was accompanied by photos and a story. The buyer could see not only who made the jewellery but also how it benefited the local community.

'Y'all wanna join me on a buying expedition to some villages north of Ubud tomorrow?'

I couldn't say yes fast enough. I'd been in the country fewer than 24 hours, and here I was being offered an adventure, one with a beautiful purpose no less. As a bonus, I would get a Matthew McConaughey look alike as my guide.

'Can y'all ride a scooter?'

I shook my head vehemently. Having seen the crazy traffic and the fact that everyone was driving on the wrong side of the road, I didn't dare contemplate risking life and limb riding a bike through such madness. He chuckled and offered to hire a Jeep in its place.

———

The morning sun rose through the hazy, humid air, its rays painting Wayan's gardens and stone statues a yellowish orange. As we escaped the craziness and traffic of Kuta, the Island of the

Gods began to live up to its name. The countryside was beautiful, a dreamscape of lush green rice paddies, ornate temples, and picturesque villages. The air smelled of frangipani flowers and incense, overlaid with the occasional waft of raw sewage and burning trash. Bali in a nutshell.

'Y'all know this here island's mainly Hindu. But they've got their own unique take on it. They call it *Agama*, kind of a combination of Buddhism and Shaivism.'

He threw me a good-natured smile and proceeded to turn off the bitumen onto a narrow winding dirt road leading up into the mountains.

'Ya see, Balinese believe in the philosophy of *Tri Hita Karana*, which is Sanskrit and kinda translates to "the three paths to wellbeing": harmony among people, harmony with nature and harmony with God.

'The first path's called *Pawongan*. It's all about tolerance and respect. Think good things, speak good things and do good things, not just for the people you know, but for, well, everyone. Unlike us Westerners, the Balinese believe we're not meant to live on our own. You wanna be truly happy? You gotta be social and you gotta give back.'

He pointed to a colourful procession winding its way through a village.

'See over there?' he said excitedly. 'The women are carrying offerings filled with food, money and flowers. They're expressing gratitude for all the bounties that the Gods provide each day.'

I'd always taken for granted our prosperity and that I'd have food to eat. I never thought about being intentionally grateful and giving some of it back.

He continued, 'Now, the second path is *Palemahan*, which is all about nature. If nature provides for you, you in turn have to repay this debt by doing your small part to preserve it. You cut down a tree here, you gotta do a proper ritual, then replace it with another tree.'

I was astounded by the idea that such deep respect for nature was ingrained into their faith.

'And finally, there's *Parhyangan*, our relationship with God. It's the biggie. They reckon when your inner world's sorted, the outer world reflects all that love and peace back at you. When y'all are in flow, the boundaries of work and gifts are blurred, you are living your truth.'

'So is that what you do?'

'Ah sure do try. It may seem to some like I'm the generous one, like I'm the giver, but by helping people, by sharing love and kindness I receive so much more in return.'

I looked at him with admiration. This was a completely different way of approaching the work-life balance. I vowed to take the philosophy on board.

We finally arrived at a tiny village near the top of the mountain. As we climbed out of the Jeep, we were greeted by a petite elegant Balinese lady in a traditional white and yellow dress. Her serene face was framed by dark hair pulled back into a neat bun. She radiated joy when she saw us.

'That there's Ni Luh. Don't she look happier than a dead pig in the sunshine?'

I shook my head. 'Seriously, Ash, I'm never gonna get used to your bizarre southern sayings.'

We wandered past half a dozen huts, dodging mangy dogs, scrawny chickens and skinny brown kids with beaming white smiles. Women walked past, balancing impossibly huge baskets on their heads. Incense sticks burned outside each building, wafting scented smoke over colourful offerings in little woven baskets. A small monkey picked over the offerings. Bali was full of surprises.

We reached the centre of the village, where there was a raised wooden platform covered by a thatched roof. It was bubbling with chatter and laughter. There were dozens of villagers seated there, each working on different parts of the bracelets. They smiled and called out, 'Selamat pagi'—good morning in Balinese. Everyone seemed abundantly peaceful.

Ni Luh beamed. 'Please, you come to see the school.' She turned to me. 'Ash buy jewellery, we make money. Families can now pay for kids' education fees. We are very thankful for him. He has spirit of *Pawongan* in his heart.'

As we walked in the door, 20 small faces lit up when they spotted Ash. After receiving a nod from their teacher, the children jumped off their seats and rushed towards him, wrapping their skinny arms around the big American's legs. They giggled with excitement. He laughed, bent down, tousled the hair of some and hugged them back. It was a touching moment.

My eyes burned with unshed tears. I wondered how it was possible that these people could be so happy with so little when I was often unhappy and had so much. Maybe poverty really was a matter of perspective. Their homes were simple, their meals were rice-based and the kids had no plastic toys, TVs or electricity, but they were rich in community, kindness and love. It was all they seemed to need. I thought back to the countless hours I'd spent on the treadmill trying to get rid of my muffin top. Damn, these people have probably never even *tasted* muffins, let alone had to deal with one protruding over their waistband.

I spent the next five days with Ash travelling through iridescent green rice paddies and up to remote mountain villages. By the time we arrived back at Wayan's place, my worldview had been turned upside down, which was ironic given I was holidaying on the 'down' side of the world. When it was time to say goodbye to my mentor and new friend, he picked me up in a big bear hug and swung me round like a ragdoll before placing me gently on the ground.

'Listen honey, a chicken's eyes may not be that far apart, but they still got sense enough to get the hell outta the rain.'

I looked at him, confused.

'The world's a big place. Time for you to set it on fire. Stop standing in the rain complainin' you're gettin' wet.'

And then he was gone.

Suddenly, I was alone once again. But I refused to dwell on it, instead choosing to go for a run and embrace my happy place. As I jogged past swanky resorts, massage ladies rubbing oil into burnt sun worshippers and beach bars full of tourists drinking brightly coloured cocktails, part of me ached to flop on a beanbag, order a Bintang and join them. But another part of me now felt compelled to do something more meaningful. Thanks Ash! The question was, what? Then it hit me. Why not put a care package together for Ni Luh's school? Perfect! I remembered Ash's words about the giver also being the receiver and the importance of true generosity. I recalled him explaining the Balinese didn't make offerings to their Gods as a form of barter but rather as a selfless action, a gesture of gratitude for everything they already had. I decided that's what I needed to do.

I detoured off the beach and straight into the heart of Kuta's 'let's bag a bargain' territory. As soon as I hit the street, a myriad sights and sounds assaulted me. I wove precariously around stalls filled with throngs of fellow tourists haggling to save 50 cents on a t-shirt. All distractions. I had a mission now, a purpose. That's when I spotted the stationery shop across the road. Looking for a gap in the traffic, I stepped off the curb.

I heard somebody yell, followed by a scream. Then I felt my body twist in the air just before my head slammed down onto the pavement. The world went black. And it stayed that way until I felt a gentle hand on my arm and a voice that sounded exactly like Sandy from Grease ask, 'Are you okay?'

Noises and smells flooded back to me in waves; car horns, motorbike engines, a hot pavement reeking of petrol. I squinted and looked around. People were crowded above me. I lay sprawled half on my belly, half on my side. I fought my way out of a deep fog and realised belatedly I was the one who had screamed. But why? Pushing myself onto my elbows with considerable effort, I noticed blood everywhere. Nearby, two girls were lying on the road next to a motorbike on its side. My brain struggled to piece it together. I must have looked the wrong way before stepping off the curb. Oh God, what have I done?

I rose shakily to my feet and staggered to the sidewalk, desperate to escape the carnage and chaos. I felt hands support me and heard yelling as someone held out a sarong. A woman pointed at the ground. I looked. One of my baby blue running shoes was now soaked in blood and there were chunks of flesh clinging to the laces. Strangely, there was no pain. I felt my head. There was a big bump but no blood. Concussion was fogging my brain. Where was the blood coming from? Then I saw it, a ragged wound the size of a tennis ball gouged out of my left calf, skin and flesh hanging loosely around it. *Damn*, I thought, *I've ruined my favourite pair of blue runners.* I sank down, nauseated. I carefully wrapped the proffered sarong around the injury. From my army days I knew I had to apply a tight bandage to stop the bleeding, but I also wanted to cover the wound to keep it clean and make it disappear. Looking at it was making me feel faint. Surrounding me was a sea of concerned faces. A kind Balinese man tried pulling me to my feet, but I resisted. From somewhere above me, I heard Sandy's voice again. I looked up and saw three blonde-haired, blue-eyed girls. Aussies!

'Don't stress, sweetheart, we'll help you.'

Relief washed over me as they helped me up. I collapsed into the safety of their arms.

Lying on the table in the Balinese doctor's office, I watched as he injected local anaesthetic into my leg. The sight of the needle made me ill. I squeezed Sandy's hand—she was really Becky from Sydney—and together we watched the doctor clean the gaping wound and stitch back the remaining skin and flesh to cover the hole. The doctor handed me antibiotics and painkillers and warned, 'Your leg do no good here. You need leave Bali now. You go home.'

By the time I hobbled to Denpasar Airport that night, my leg and foot had swollen dramatically. I tried to get my left shoe on but failed. The bloody psychic was right! Her premonition had nothing to do with a leg press.

I thought about the irony of my situation. The hole in my soul had begun to mend thanks to Ash and the happiness I'd experienced in the Balinese villages, but now it had been replaced by a physical one—in my leg, no less! I'd asked the universe for an adventure and a life-changing experience but had forgotten the old adage, *be careful what you wish for*. The sensible thing to do would have been to book a flight home, back to my family and Canada where there was fully covered medical care. But I've rarely been accused of being sensible. And so I crossed my fingers and took a chance on a far more uncertain future instead.

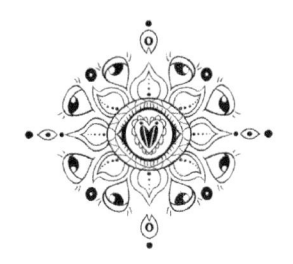

CHAPTER FOURTEEN
Life Is But a Dream

Alice: Would you tell me, please, which way I ought to go from here?
Cheshire Cat: That depends a good deal on where you want to get to.
~ Lewis Carroll

The plane banked over Sydney Harbour, the sparkling waters framed by a stunning coastline of beaches, sandstone cliffs and sandy coves. The rays of the morning sun flashed off the white-tiled sails of the Opera House, greeting me with a wink as if to say, 'You made it.' I was finding it hard to fully appreciate the moment. I'd just spent six hours watching my leg swell to epic proportions. It looked like an overstuffed sausage ready to burst from its skin, and despite the painkillers, it was throbbing with pain. In addition, I was flanked by three drunken Irish backpackers making the most of the complimentary booze.

Normally I would have joined them, but I was worried about anything hampering my already-precarious balance. It was easy to forgive the Irish trio for being boisterous, however. They were the ones responsible for me being on the plane, having literally scooped me off the floor of Denpasar Airport ten hours earlier. At the time I'd been in real trouble, hobbling through the concourse, weighed down by my oversized backpack, wearing only one shoe. As I reached the check-in line, I toppled over, and the boys valiantly came to my rescue. It seemed like rescuers travelled in packs of three in Bali.

'Fer Chrissake, lass, whatcha doin'? You can barely walk.'

'Had a fight with a motorbike and lost,' I groaned. I rolled over on the cool tiles and looked into three sunburnt, freckled faces. 'But I'm not letting a mere flesh wound stop me! I'm going to Australia.'

They chuckled as they helped me up. 'You stick with us lass. We'll look after you.'

And they were true to their word. They carried my bag out of Sydney airport and helped me board a bus destined for Coogee Beach, a laid-back suburb known for its surf. On arrival, the boys were keen to see the sights, but the only sight I wanted to see was the inside of a doctor's office. Liam, aka Big Red, the gentle giant of the trio, opted to stay and help me hop to the nearest medical clinic. The doctor there took one look at my swollen appendage and sent me straight to hospital. He explained I had severe trauma and possibly a severed tendon, in which case immediate surgery was required. So off I hopped to the emergency room at The Prince of Wales Hospital, fearing the worst.

On closer examination of my wound, the doctors there had better news for me. While the motorbike pedal had caused extensive tissue damage, it had narrowly missed my tendon and I didn't require surgery. They were duly impressed by the Balinese doctor's handiwork. Within minutes they had replaced my dressings and advised me to rest, ice and elevate—with a stern warning not to swim in the ocean.

Hours later when we returned to the backpackers, it wasn't hard for the boys to convince me that the best place to recover was the Coogee Beach Hotel. Lots of ice, plenty of chairs to rest and elevate my leg on and, of course, medicinal Guinness. Connor and Aiden had some exciting news.

'I got us a job, startin' tomorrow,' said Connor.

'Unless it's as a one-legged pole dancer, best count me out.'

'Na, yer'll be great, no legs required,' assured Aiden.

'What have you got us into now you eejit?' Liam was sceptical.

'We're sellin' protection,' Connor grinned. 'Protection for leather that is, shining' shoes at the Sydney Royal Easter Show.' He raised his glass. 'Here's to a profitable two weeks.'

With a boy on either side, I hopped into the showgrounds the next morning, not knowing what to expect. I was wearing only one of my favourite blue runners as my foot was still too swollen to squeeze into the other. The Royal Easter Show was a highly anticipated annual event, an eclectic mix of agricultural extravaganza, carnival rides and pavilions full of prizewinning chickens, flowers and fruitcakes. A world where the city mingled with the country.

We passed the show ring, where manic border collies, directed by the whistles of Akubra-clad farmers, were rounding up small flocks of sheep. Jillaroos and Jackaroos strutted about wearing spit-polished RM Williams boots, while big-gutted, skinny-legged 'carnies' waited to open their rides, patiently smoking their Winnie Blues. We finally arrived at the livestock pavilion and found a stall advertising 'Bob's Best Ever Beeswax – World's Best Leather Protection'.

Shirley, Bob's cousin, was running the show. She herded us into four seats behind wooden boxes. Our job was to convince passers-by to place their boots on our boxes so we could demonstrate just how amazing Bob's beeswax was. Another group of young foreigners, all recruited from a backpacker accommodation, were already set up next to us. They looked on with amusement.

'Well, this should be some craic.' Liam rubbed his hands together. 'First one to make a hundred bucks is buyin' tonight.'

Two hours later my three Irish mates were done, their little pots of protection still unopened in their hands.

'This is fockin' crap. Fockin' bees need to stick to making fockin' honey.' Liam slammed his pot onto the box. 'I say we go find the beer tent.'

On the other hand, I was smashing it. Consummate saleswoman that I was, I'd already sold a dozen tins of Bob's Best Ever Beeswax. After going door to door in sub-arctic conditions, this was a walk in the park for me. As the money rolled in, I whispered a silent prayer of thanks to the coupon cult, Italian stallion Tony and good old God with an R for teaching me the fine art of selling. For the next two weeks, I worked 12-hour shifts, polishing furiously. Each night at the pub I'd gleefully display fistfuls of cash to the boys and yell out, 'First round's on me, lads!' Sure, it wasn't exactly what I had in mind after leaving Bali—I wasn't living a life of purpose or setting the world on fire by shining shoes—but at least I was resting my leg all day and making good money while doing it. My real dream was to get the hell out of the city. I wanted to look a kangaroo in the eye and dive into the red dust of the outback.

After I finished my last day of work and shouted a last round of Guinness at the Coogee Hotel, we all decided it was time to head north and follow the sun to the fabled surf and hippie mecca of Byron Bay.

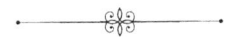

Byron was everything we'd hoped it would be: stunning white sand beaches, dazzlingly brilliant blue water, bronzed Aussie surfers and pods of playful dolphins. The famous Cape Byron lighthouse marked the most easterly point in Australia and was the perfect spot to watch migrating humpbacks on their winter pilgrimage from Antarctica to the Great Barrier Reef.

The ocean called out to me, and it frustrated me no end that I was still unable to answer it. Just before leaving Sydney, an overzealous doctor had removed my stitches prematurely, and the wound in my leg had gone from bad to horrific, developing into a yellow ulcer surrounded by decaying flesh. It smelled even worse than it looked. I tried to hold it together with Steri-Strips and Band-Aids, but it wasn't working. Worst of all, my travel insurance had run out and my medical costs were mounting. The doctor I'd seen in Byron for treatment had warned me: if it didn't heal soon I'd need a skin graft at best, an amputation at worst. I came to the sad realisation I'd pushed my luck as far as I could. It was time to go home, give up on my dream of seeing the outback and have my leg properly attended to.

Fate intervened that night in the form of a cute Irish redhead named Frances. It seemed to me an unfortunate name for such a stunning girl. We exchanged stories. I told her about my leprous leg, and she told me about a magical place in far north Queensland called the Whitsunday Islands, located within the Great Barrier Reef. Frances was on her way back to Ireland after sailing around the islands and offered to give me her medical insurance card. All I had to do was pretend to be her. I knew it was wrong, but hey, desperate times called for desperate measures.

Each time the boys and I travelled north, making our way from one beachside paradise to the next, I would check into a local doctor's office, presenting 'my' medical insurance card. While the guys partied it up on the Gold Coast and enjoyed stunning vistas of endless beaches on their 4WD trip around Fraser Island, the largest sand island in the world, my vistas were of dead flesh being cut away from my festering wound and bandages being reapplied to the contours of my calf. It was a sobering experience. My goal was to do everything I could to close the damn hole and go sailing around the Whitsundays. It had now been exactly a month since Liam, Connor, Aiden, and

I had been travelling together, and our next stop would finally be Airlie Beach, gateway to the Whitsunday Islands.

From Hervey Bay, we endured another long overnight bus ride. I dozed on and off in the front seat until I was awakened by the first rays of the morning sun. We crested a hill covered in eucalypts and jungle. Below lay a glittering expanse of turquoise water framed by islands, anchored yachts and a marina full of boats painted gold by the sun. Lush tropical hills spilled into a series of calm aquamarine bays fringed by coconut palms. *Oh my, this is Airlie?* It took my breath away. I looked up and whispered a silent prayer.

'Please God, let me stay here for a while.'

We checked into the backpackers and, hey presto, there it was, a sign from above. Quite literally a sign, taped above the desk announcing 'Cleaner Wanted'. Paddy, the Irish owner, explained it was three hours a day in exchange for $30 and a bed in the eight-person staff dorm. I accepted immediately. After stowing my gear in the staff quarters, I headed out to find a medical clinic.

'Name please.'

'Ka...I mean Frances.' I presented the receptionist with my purloined insurance card. So far so good. I joined the rest of the patients in the small waiting room. A short time later a GP emerged from one of the consultation rooms and called the next patient. My jaw dropped. He was gorgeous, tanned and fit with rugged good looks, dark wavy hair and a sexy Scottish accent.

'Frances?' He glanced around. 'Frances?'

I came to my senses and realised he was calling me. I jumped up and hobbled towards him. He smiled warmly, introduced himself and ushered me into his office with a wave of his hand. Damn, did I really have to show him my disgusting leg? I thought about making up another excuse as to why I was seeing him.... Diarrhoea? Pap smear? No, you idiot, those were even worse.

'So, Frances,' he enquired, 'how canna help ye?'

I explained my predicament, saying I'd been to countless doctors while travelling up the coast in a bid to heal my festering wound.

'I've had a lot of conflicting advice about how to treat it, but nothing seems to be working.'

'Okay, well let's have a wee look, shall we?'

With deft fingers he began taking off the dressing covering the unsightly hole in my leg. My heartbeat quickened, partly because it always did when my wound was revealed and partly because he had now grasped my leg in his capable hands and had gently lifted it to get a better view of the injury.

'Ah now, ya see lassie, that's nae good,' he said softly. 'But nae ta worry. I can help ye. The good news is, I've studied tropical medicine, and ah know all about these types of ulcers. I can get ye sorted, but I'll need tae see ye every day.'

I almost laughed. Seriously, was Doctor McGorgeous telling me I'd have to see him daily? I could hardly believe my luck.

'Are ye able to stop here awhile, Frances?'

Only for the rest of my life, I thought but instead replied, 'Sure. I'm planning on staying put for quite a while.'

'Ah'm verra pleased ta hear that, Frances.'

I watched his hands as he skilfully cut away bits of my rotting flesh and then cleaned and treated the wound before re-dressing it snugly. As I half-floated, half-limped out of the office, he gave me a reassuring wink.

'So I'll be seein' ye tomorrow. We'll have ye good as new in no time.'

No rush, I thought. *No rush at all.*

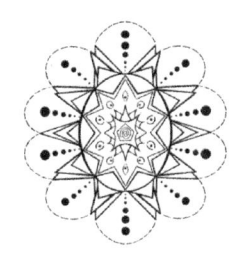

CHAPTER FIFTEEN
Fate, Destiny or Karma

I don't know if we each have a destiny or if we are all just floatin' around accidental-like on a breeze, but I...I think maybe it's both, maybe both is happenin' at the same time.
~ Forrest Gump

My new life in Airlie Beach was now in full swing. Each morning I'd jump out of bed at six to start cleaning. I was finished by nine, and my roomies teased me while I gussied myself up for my daily doctor's appointment.

'Off to see Dr Sean Connery?'

'Yes, my future husband,' I'd reply jokingly.

Fortunately—or unfortunately, depending on how you looked at the situation—the wound started to heal. And although I knew he was well above my pay grade, I couldn't help but flirt with my sexy Scottish doctor. He was funny, kind and patient, and we hit it off. I found myself looking forward to my appointment, and after it was finished, I'd spend the rest of the day eagerly awaiting my next visit.

Meanwhile, the Irish boys had decided to continue on their path of mischievous mayhem and head north to Cairns. I hated saying goodbye to my lovable rogues—they'd been my guardian angels since my arrival in Oz. After they left I sat by the beach, looking at the expanse of the Coral Sea. I'd arrived in Bali lost, confused and alone. Then I'd met Ash, the Sandy trio and the Irish lads and collected a bagful of extraordinary experiences. Now here I was, a solo traveller again. This time, however, the prospect of being alone no longer scared me. Hah! Feel the fear and do it anyway. Thanks Susan Jeffers.

Over the next month I attended the clinic religiously, and my wound healed. I was simultaneously relieved and distraught. Yes, the good doctor had closed the hole in my leg, but my yearning for him had opened another gaping hole—in my heart. As I walked out of his office following my final appointment, he tenderly rested a hand on my shoulder, looked down at me and said, 'Mind yae look the right way before crossing the road.'

I smiled, and for a moment we stood gazing at each other. He began to say something, then stopped himself. It seemed he was as disappointed as I was that our medical relationship was ending and that I now no longer had a legitimate excuse to see him again.

Later that day my friends at the backpackers decided we should go to Hog's Breath Café to celebrate the miracle of my cured leg—not that anyone ever needed an excuse to party in Airlie Beach. Jimmy Buffett's 'Margaritaville' was playing in the background of the packed bar. I glanced around, and my gaze landed on a familiar face. It was none other than my gorgeous Scottish doctor. At that instant, he looked straight at me. I froze. *Oh my God, he's seen me.* I looked away only to have my friends crash into my back.

'What the hell girl! You're causing a traffic jam.'

I stole another glance in his direction, and he was smiling and waving.

'Frances!'

I looked around, mystified as to who he was waving at. But of course—it was me.

The music drifted on the warm tropical breeze, enveloping me in Jimmy Buffett's iconic lyrics about Margaritaville and searching for a shaker of salt. I wondered if Frances was the woman to blame or if it was my own damn fault.

My heart beat wildly. I didn't know whether to stay or bolt. Was this fate? Destiny? What the hell, I decided, feel the fear, do it anyway. I approached him.

'Well now, look at ye, walking normal again.'

'I've been working on normal for quite a while now,' I replied, 'but I've had lots of help from a very clever doctor.'

He laughed. 'Aye, but now I'm nae your doctor anymore, right luv?'

He raised his glass. I toasted him back. Did he just call me luv?

We sat at the bar, deep in conversation. Occasionally we would be interrupted by one of my co-workers drunkenly urging us to join them. Upon hearing his accent, they'd whisper into my ear for all the world to hear, 'It's your hot Scottish doctor!' I was mortified. But he didn't seem too fazed by the fact I'd obviously spoken about him at great length. Over a bottle or two of ice-cold chardy we proceeded to get to know each other on a more intimate level. At least now he was gazing longingly into my eyes, rather than at the hole in my leg. He brushed a stray hair away from my face and murmured, 'Aye Frances, what do you say we leave Margaritaville for somewhere quieter?'

I couldn't quite believe it. Yet another man who I thought was unattainable was wanting to take me home, only this time I didn't have to buy him.

I just wished he'd stop calling me Frances.

I showed up for work at six sharp the following morning, looking a tad ruffled, and still dressed in my clothes from the night before. Paddy called me into his office.

'Someone looks like they didn't get much sleep last night.'

I blushed, unable to hide my inner glow.

'Well now, none of my business,' he grinned. 'I've got a surprise for you.' He paused for dramatic effect.

'*What* already?' I hated being left hanging.

'There's a yacht leaving this morning for a five-day cruise around the islands. Skipper's a mate of mine. He needs an extra hostie to help him out. I said you'd be perfect for the job.'

'Really? Oh my God, thank you!'

'My niece is here for a few weeks. She'll cover for you.'

I skipped around the desk and gave him a big hug.

Paddy patted my back impatiently. 'Best you hurry now, all hands on deck by 0800.'

Bolting out of the office I yelled, 'If a hot Scot drops by, tell him I'll be back.'

He raised his eyebrows and nodded.

I was the luckiest girl in the world. I'd spent a night of abandon with Doctor McGorgeous and now I'd been offered a free trip around the Whitsundays. To top it off, my leg was healed and I could finally swim in an Australian ocean. Euphoric didn't even come close to describing the happiness I felt.

I threw some clothes into my bag and tore down to the marina. When I finally found the yacht, I laughed out loud. The name stencilled boldly on the stern: *Destiny*. Of course it was. Howie, the skipper, greeted me like an old friend. He was a jovial, heavy-set older man with sunburnt cheeks. He introduced me to his petite Vietnamese wife An'h, who also happened to be his chief cook, provisioner and deckie. They outlined my duties and gave me a quick tour of the yacht. Shortly afterwards the guests arrived and we were ready to hoist sail and set off.

We crossed the deep blue waters of the Whitsunday Passage as we tacked towards our first anchorage, Nara Inlet on Hook Island. Steep, tree-covered mountains and colourful reefs lined both sides of the narrow waterway. In essence, it was a tropical version of a fjord. Every now and again a turtle popped its head up, as if curious to see what the splashing was all about, before dipping below the surface a few seconds later. It was so overwhelmingly beautiful I almost cried. I dove into the clear, warm waters and straight into a school of brightly striped fish. This was the moment I'd been waiting for. I was in heaven.

That night I lay on the deck, the yacht rolling gently on a small swell. I gazed at the Milky Way splashed across the heavens in all its glory. Everything was falling into place: a new man, a new leg and a new life. Frances was right, this place was every bit of amazing—and best of all not an icicle in sight. The next few days flew by as we sailed from one beautiful anchorage to the next. By the time we reached the jewel in the Whitsundays' crown, stunning Whitehaven Beach, I was a veteran sailor, tanned golden by the tropical sun. I was as handy on the winches, ropes and mainsail as I was cooking in the galley. After laying anchor, I once again dove into the clear blue waters and swam to shore, luxuriating in the soft, powder-white silica sand. No wonder it was voted one of the top beaches in the world.

My thoughts eventually drifted back to my Scottish doctor. Despite having an incredible time sailing I was anxious to return to the man who I'd never thought in a million lifetimes would choose someone like me. I felt bad for leaving without a word and disappearing for a week. He was probably wondering what the hell happened to me. I spent my last night wide awake on the deck of *Destiny*, fantasising about our imminent reunion, wondering where we would end up living, the day of our wedding, how many kids we'd have...ah, life is but a dream within a dream.

We arrived back at Abel Point Marina just as dusk was falling. I felt on top of the world as I strolled to the backpackers where Paddy's niece was manning the front desk. We introduced ourselves, and I asked if any mail had arrived while I was away.

'No mail, unless you count the cute bloke with the Scottish accent who came by looking for Frances.'

I clapped my hands, 'Yay!'

Paddy's niece bit her lip 'Yeah, but…I told him there was no Frances here, that maybe she left. He seemed a bit sad.'

My happy bubble popped. 'Wait, what? No!'

'Sorry. When Paddy got back, he said you were Frances, which I thought was weird, 'cause I thought you were Kat. Hope I didn't mess things up.'

I hardly paused to drop my bag in my room before sprinting up the hill to his apartment, a hundred thoughts swirling in my head. So I'd lied about my name, slept with him, then disappeared for nearly a week. He'd understand, right? After all, he was my destiny. I reached his apartment, made a futile attempt to tame my salt-crusted hair, caught my breath, then knocked.

When he opened the door, I threw my arms wide and yelled, 'Surprise!'

'Frances?'

'Actually…uh…no, but I am really me. And there was this last-minute sailing job—'

He tried to interject but I was determined to finish what I had to say.

'—that was too good to turn down. I didn't have time to let you know, but I'm back now.'

I squeezed past him into his living room. 'And I couldn't stop thinking about—'

I stopped mid-sentence. The table in his living room had been set for two: candles, wine, flowers. My heart melted. How did he know? Then the bathroom door opened and a blonde bombshell wearing a sexy black dress and strappy stilettos strode out. To say it was an awkward moment would be an understatement. She looked at me, I looked at her, and then we both looked at the man of our dreams.

'Ah, Sally, this is Frances...wait, no it's not. What's your real name?'

'Kat,' I groaned. 'It's Kat, I'm sorry, I've been trying to tell you.'

I glanced back at the Claudia Schiffer lookalike and knew instantly who the winner of this chicken dinner would be. I turned and bolted out the door, trailing humiliation and embarrassment in my wake, along with shards of my shattered dreams.

What do you do when reality bites, especially when that reality is completely at odds with your dreams? You run away as fast as you can. I hurtled down the hill, past the backpackers, past Hog's Breath and the medical centre, until I finally reached the water's edge and collapsed onto the sand. As I lay there heaving, once again staring up at the Milky Way, I covered my face with my hands, attempting to block out all the 'if onlys'. *Did you really expect him to marry you when he didn't even know your name?* I thought about the absurdity of the situation and laughed until tears poured down my face. *Oh God, you fool, what the hell were you thinking Frances!* I returned to the backpackers and crawled into my top bunk, reminiscing about my family and friends on the other side of the world until I started to nod off. Maybe it was time to move on.

The next morning as I gazed into my cup, desperately trying to read my tea leaves, I thought back over the whole crazy situation. Surely things happened for a reason; it wasn't all just random chance, right? Maybe life is like one of those choose-your-own-adventure books, where each time you make a decision it results in a radically different outcome. If I'd decided not to take the yacht trip that day, would I still be with the hot Scot? I concluded the point was moot. You couldn't argue with reality. I needed to radically accept it. If I wanted better tomorrows it was best not to dwell on the 'what ifs' and instead focus on more constructive goals, like getting another job to top up my adventure funds. What was it someone once said? 'Worrying about tomorrow doesn't change tomorrow. But it does change today—and not for the better.'

I started my cleaning rounds, and Paddy waved me into his office. He had another surprise for me. It was a part-time job with a friend of his who owned a boarding house up the hill.

'John's a little eccentric but a good guy, and between here and there you'll have a full-time gig.'

'Oh, great,' I muttered.

'Ah lass, sorry to hear about your doctor.'

What the hell! Were there no secrets around here? Paddy wrapped me in a fatherly hug.

'I always say, never trust a man who wears a skirt.'

I shrugged despondently. 'Guess it just wasn't my destiny.'

John's 'house' turned out to be a two-storey white concrete mansion—hence its local nickname, the 'White House'. It had seen better days. I knocked on the door, avoiding peeling strips of paint.

'Come in, come in,' John said exuberantly.

He was wearing cotton wrap-around fisherman's pants, Mala beads around his neck and a loose long-sleeved shirt. In a strong English accent, he explained that he'd just returned to Oz after spending time visiting the Dalai Lama's residence in India.

'I've been inspired by his spirituality. I want to turn this place into a serene oasis to calm the mind and soothe the soul.'

He walked me around the dilapidated house, outlining his ideas for each room with enthusiasm. He flung open a bathroom door to describe the underwater mural he envisaged being painted there, and we were immediately confronted by a naked, blonde surfie-looking dude stepping out of the shower. I tried and failed not to stare at his rock-hard body as droplets of water dripped towards his nether regions.

The surfie quickly grabbed a towel, wrapped it around his waist and gave me a lopsided grin.

'Ah, Trevor, meet Kat. Kat, meet Trevor,' John said without a hint of embarrassment.

When I forced my gaze to lift from his torso I noticed a gentleness in his blue eyes. They were framed by an angular face, a strong jaw and full lips. Trevor shook my hand and introduced himself very formally as 'Trevor Donovan from Jrudgerie'.

Jrudgerie? Where the hell was that?

John interrupted my thoughts.

'Kat's my new interior decorator, aren't you darling?'

Mmm, right, I thought, nodding my head in agreement. I had no idea how to be an interior decorator but I was willing to give it a red-hot go. As if sensing my apprehension, Trevor gave me a playful smile. He was no Scottish doctor, but he radiated charm and charisma.

John, sensing the need to highlight the importance of the occasion, flung his arms wide and announced, 'Kat is going to transform our world.'

And I did, only it wasn't John's.

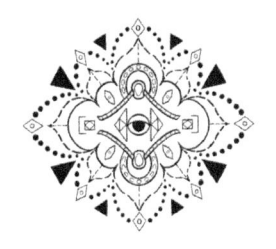

CHAPTER SIXTEEN
Everything I Never Wanted

*Knowing what you like doesn't mean
you should only like what you know
~ Erin Hanson*

The White House…dilapidated haven for lost souls, itinerant Aussie travellers, idealistic self-help gurus and young Canadian backpackers with broken dreams. It was the opposite of its more famous namesake in America, both in looks and in its underlying political and moral spectrum. Although John's vision for the place didn't quite match the reality, I soon found myself loving the vibe there. My only stumbling block was my experience in the artistic and painting department. I was no Michelangelo. Truth was, I used to skip out on art classes at school.

I stared at the blank bathroom walls and wondered how the hell I was going to paint the magnificent Great Barrier Reef mural that my new boss had envisaged splashed across them. I started arranging the pots of blue, green, red, and yellow paint across the floor, rolled up my sleeves and kicked off my underwater masterpiece. Coral? Easy. Colourful reef fish? No problem. Clamshells? Piece of cake. Eight hours later I was done. Paint-splattered and triumphant, I stepped back to admire my creation and knew immediately it was a complete and utter disaster.

As I sat miserably on the toilet seat, head in hands, I pictured future residents wondering who the hell was responsible for the unglorified mess surrounding them. Just then, Trevor, the golden-haired surfer boy, walked in and offered to help. The memory of him naked in the same bathroom days earlier popped into my head. I smiled, and he smiled back. I prayed he couldn't guess I was having a morally ambiguous déjà vu moment. It turned out Trevor was not just a cute guy but also an undefeated amateur boxer from the outback and, as fate would have it, a qualified painter and decorator. I was saved! We spent the rest of the night fixing up the mural together.

Trevor—or Trev, as any Aussie would call him—represented pretty much everything I never wanted in a guy. I'd always pictured myself with a sophisticated, sharply dressed man—tall, dark, handsome, with underlying rugged tones. The Scottish doctor checked the right boxes, however Trev was the antithesis of this. I'd never seen him wearing a shirt or proper shoes, just a pair of board shorts, thongs and shades. He was easy-going, chilled out, a bit on the wild side...and he smoked pot! He was certainly not someone who would normally be on my radar. But over time he grew on me, kinda like a yeast infection, one you know you shouldn't scratch but do anyway. On the days I worked at the White House he'd stroll out of his room in a pair of loose boxers, smile and offer me a Vegemite sandwich. I'd politely decline—I couldn't stand the stuff! In fact, I couldn't ever imagine a time where I'd be able to stomach the vile black yeast extract Aussies loved so much. But it was sweet of him to offer all the same.

We were both backpackers working our way around Australia. Turned out that, although he surfed, he was an outback country boy from a small town snuggled deep in the interior of New South Wales. He started asking me to stay for 'tea', which on many occasions ended up being the fish he'd caught that day. We chatted easily and had one of those rare connections where the world could have exploded and we wouldn't have noticed.

Everything about him enthralled me. I even loved watching him eat, the way he methodically and slowly chewed his food, the slight clicking of his once-broken jaw, his impeccable table manners. Best of all, he owned the entire cassette tape collection of Prince, of whom I was a die-hard fan. He knew every word to every song. I found myself being reeled in, hook, line and sinker, just like the fish on my plate.

The clincher came when he invited me out on our first official 'date'. Trev had three sisters and was very familiar with the world of girls. Well aware I was living out of a backpack, he chose not to buy me flowers and champagne but instead showed up with a black-and-white polka dot dress exactly my size and some foam stick rollers he'd found at the second-hand shop. I was touched and just a tad bemused when he offered to give me an 'up do' and curl my hair before whisking me off to his favourite restaurant. It was the nicest, most thoughtful thing a man had ever done for me!

His favourite restaurant turned out to be the Hog's Breath Café, a place I'd been studiously avoiding since my Highland fling. As we walked past the bar area and made our way to the rear of the restaurant where the dining room was, my nervousness escalated. I stole a quick glance around, half expecting to see Frances' former lover canoodling with his supermodel but he was nowhere to be seen. Phew! Our table on the back verandah overlooked the sheltered waters of Pioneer Bay. Lights from dozens of anchored yachts swayed in the darkness, creating a kind of shimmering mini-Milky Way. Overhead, 'The Piña Colada' song wafted through hidden speakers. I couldn't help but sing along to the catchy lyrics, wondering if this man in front of me was the love I was looking for and if we'd plan our escape. Trev grinned and sang along with me.

It was very romantic and kind of awkward at the same time. But a few glasses of wine helped us both relax. Trev had the most incredible eyes, light blue, playful and full of life, and I found myself falling into them as he regaled me with stories of his childhood in a small outback town. This sweet, rugged guy was a walking contradiction—boxer, feminist, country boy, surfer—all rolled into one incredibly sexy package. At one point he reached across the table and gently laid his hand on mine.

'You know, I was supposed to be on Daydream Island tonight with a friend. But I chose to be here with you instead.'

I squeezed his hand in return. 'Trev Donovan, as my Aunt Kath would say, you are a dish, even if you are a bit of a player. But thank you for making me feel special.'

Walking home hand in hand after dinner, we stopped beneath the walls of the White House and kissed for the first time.

Uh oh, I think I'm seriously falling for this guy, my wine-addled brain whispered to me. I hoped to God the reverse was true.

As if in reply to my internal conversation, Trev held me in his arms and swayed gently as he hummed the last bars of the Pina Colada song. 'Are you the lady I've been looking for?'

'Yes,' I murmured back, 'I will come with you and escape.'

We laughed and waltzed our way to his room, singing the rest of the song together.

The next morning, as I lay there beside him in a hazy bliss, I began thinking to myself, *What is it about the craziness of love that makes life so unpredictable and yet so magical?* Trev opened my eyes to the possibility that perhaps I'd been pursuing the wrong dream all this time, that maybe what I needed and what I wanted were two very different things. He made me rethink my idea of happiness. Our connection was based on enjoying the simpler things in life, it wasn't fancy cars, fine dining, flashy hotels and superficial good looks. In fact, I was fast discovering that true love wasn't about getting what I wanted all the time, but more about loving what I already had. And Trev was a living lesson in how to be selfless, kind, content and happy no matter the circumstances. I found the whole situation refreshing and endearing.

After two inseparable months together we decided it was time to depart the paradise of Airlie and set off on a new adventure. Trev was the proud owner of a beige '78 dual-cab Toyota Land Cruiser, a classic Aussie outback 4WD. I was nearly as turned on by his wheels as I was by his washboard abs. The truck sported a bench seat, an independent battery running power to the lights and a small fan in the 'bedroom' in the back—a comfy double bed with a large mosquito net hanging over it. The rear of the truck was surrounded by a protective metal cage with canvas roll-up sides. It was built high enough that you could almost stand as you dressed. There was a snorkel for deep river crossings, a winch to pull you out of muddy holes, surfboard racks, two spare tyres, fishing rods, and a gun for hunting pigs. He also had a large esky to keep the food cold and the drinks even colder. Not exactly five-star, but pretty damn close for a travelling outback home.

We hit the road, heading for Cairns and the tropical far north. Adventure was calling and I was ready and willing to take on the challenge, even if it meant confronting pretty much all of Australia's most deadly critters along the way. Spiders, snakes, crocs, box jellyfish, blue-ringed octopus, feral pigs, sharks, even a giant flightless bird with dinosaur feet called a cassowary that apparently roamed the rainforests of the north in search of backpackers to disembowel. Trev also told me about drop bears, a mutant version of the cuddly koala, which dropped out of trees onto unsuspecting hikers and tore them to pieces with razor-sharp teeth. Holy hell, in Canada we only had big things you could see coming, like moose and bears and very cold weather. Trev eventually admitted the drop bear story was an urban myth but winked and swore the cassowary story was ridgy-didge. My eyes sparkled with excitement.

'Woohoo,' I hollered. 'Bring it on!'

'Crazy Canadian.'

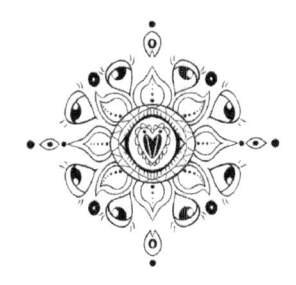

CHAPTER SEVENTEEN
No More Itch to Scratch

Life is not made up by the breaths we take,
but the moments that take our breath away.
~ Maya Angelou

Thus began our trip of a lifetime around Australia, barrelling down a semi-deserted highway through lush cane fields, music blaring, our 2x80 air conditioning working like a charm—two windows down, 80 km/h top speed. The humid tropical breeze swirled through the cabin and whipped my hair into a frenzy. I pressed up close to him on the bench seat, my head resting on his shoulder, his arm casually slung around me. He gently kissed the top of my head. It was one of those freeze-frame moments you remember with intense clarity and joy years later in life.

Our north Queensland road trip saw us discover treehouses, hippies, Aboriginals, and yes, real giant cassowaries in the ancient Daintree Rainforest north of Cairns. When we hit the

Northern Territory we fished for barramundi in the croc-infested Mary River and fed hordes of hungry tourists while working as cooks near Kakadu National Park. We revelled in the wide-open spaces, big skies and red dirt of the outback. We even climbed that big red rock in the middle of Australia that Aboriginals call Uluru. Our campsites were awash with kangaroos, galahs, colourful parrots, and the occasional herd of feral camels. The camels had apparently been brought over from India and Afghanistan to help with the construction of inland roads and railways in the 19th century, then left to wander when their work was done. Oh, but the one thing I found hard to swallow, literally, were the flies! Millions of them. Everywhere. They swarmed over every part of my body, in my ears, eyes, nose and mouth. They were maddening. Trev seemed completely unfazed by them. He was like one of those poor African kids in a 'Save the Children' campaign on TV, oblivious to their presence.

Every kilometre we travelled brought us closer together, but one particular incident cemented my love for him and defined why I'd fallen so crazy hard for this guy. We'd just left the Mary River and were driving down yet another dusty outback track when I noticed a burning smell. The cab began filling with smoke. I looked down. The rubber mat under my feet was on fire.

'Fire!' I screamed, stomping on the flames.

Trev screeched to a stop, jumped out, threw his seat forward, grabbed the fire extinguisher, and put the fire out before I could even make sense of what was happening. 'Damn he's good,' I said quietly to myself, and then thought, *What the hell are we going to do now?* Within minutes Trev had disconnected the second battery, found the source of the fire, rigged up some new wiring, and managed to get us back on the road. And there it was. No matter how seemingly desperate the situation, he always managed to MacGyver up a way out of it. He was rock solid, someone you could rely on in troubled times. Yes, he may not have been the tall, dark, sharply dressed man of my dreams, but maybe, just maybe, he was what I needed in my life right now. I think it was Mick Jagger who said it best when he sang we don't always get what we want all the time but if we try hard enough we just might find, we get what we need.

We clocked over 5,000 km on the road before finally making it to Darwin, Australia's northernmost city and capital of the Northern Territory. It was more of a country town on steroids than a proper city. We arrived during the build-up to the wet, aka troppo season. The intensity of the heat and humidity only served to add to the excitement of the place. Being able to immerse ourselves in the multicultural food scene after weeks of relative isolation in the outback was a joy. We ate our way through outdoor markets and cafés and quenched our thirst with icy cold beers at the Trailer Boat Club while watching the sun set over the ocean.

After stocking up on food and supplies we headed for our next destination, Litchfield National Park, the jewel in the crown of the NT's national park system. Unlike tropical north Queensland, the landscape south of Darwin was drier, more open and characterised by thousands of giant 'magnetic' termite mounds angled exactly due north to stop the critter cities from overheating. Some were a staggering four metres high—impressive indeed for an insect no bigger than a match head. Signs along the road announced *We Like Our Lizards Frilled, Not Grilled!* referring to the quirky behaviour of the unusual local inhabitants, the so-called frill-necked lizards. They had an unfortunate habit of basking on the warm road after a cold night on the outback sands and getting pancaked flat by cars.

Litchfield proved every bit as stunning as its reputation. We swam in crystal-clear pools fed by waterfalls cascading over sandstone cliffs and explored secluded creeks lined with paperbarks and pandanus. When dusk fell, we set up camp on the outskirts of the Lost City, an impressive collection of eerily eroded spires and rocky outcrops 500 million years in the making. Trev built a fire, and I prepared a hearty kangaroo stew in the camp oven—a thick cast iron pot with a heavy lid designed to cook food low and slow over hot coals. We cracked open a box of $10 Lambrusco, our favourite budget wine, and settled into our camp chairs to enjoy a spectacular view of the Milky Way.

As I lifted the lid to check on the tenderness of the roo stew, I noticed out of the corner of my eye something large, black and hairy moving towards me. I glanced to my right and saw a massive black spider rearing up on its hind legs to expose impressively large fangs. My heart stopped. The spider lunged. I froze, my brain refusing to acknowledge the reality of the situation. Where I come from, spiders run away from humans. My dad used to say, 'No need to be scared of spiders; they're a lot more scared of us than we are of them.' Apparently, none of that sensible British logic had made its way to the Land Down

Under. After overcoming my initial shock, I took off running around the fire, screaming hysterically.

Having already consumed a good half cask of Lambrusco, Trev was a touch late springing to the rescue from his chair. But, like a dedicated devotee at an Anthony Robbins seminar, he bravely ran across the hot coals to save me. He dove towards the hairy, attacking arachnid and smashed it heroically with the cardboard cask of vino. I couldn't tell from my position on the opposite side of the fire whether the spider had perished from being smothered in cheap wine or from the impact of the box. Either way, the critter was crushed. Trevor lay sprawled on the ground, groaning in pain. I helped him hobble to bed on blistered feet, scraped the corpse from the remains of the Lambrusco and soothed his pain with mugfuls of wine and cool water from the nearby creek.

The next morning, hungover and footsore, Trev admitted he was in no shape to drive. He tossed me the keys, saying, 'She's all yours baby!' I proceeded to navigate the Land Cruiser through some of the toughest terrain in the park, a monumental feat considering the number of signs warning the tracks were for experienced drivers only. Trev was duly impressed, even though at one stage I accidentally drove straight into an enormous dead tree and knocked it over. Luckily, we had a bull bar. I managed to make it to our next stop, the Daly River, with all four tyres intact and only a few minor scratches and dents to show for my amateur four-wheel driving efforts.

When we finally arrived at the caravan park, we quickly realised we were the only guests, unless you counted the resident emu. The giant, dopey bird was Trevor's shadow from the instant we pulled in. Wherever he went, it went. If Trevor went to the shower block, the emu followed. When Trev jumped in the pool, the emu dove in straight after. It was hilarious to watch and highly entertaining. Trev's affinity with animals blew my mind. If there was a two or four-legged creature in sight, Trev would quickly become besties with it.

We spent the next few days chilling on the banks of the river and exploring the surrounding bushland. Trev would set out with a rod and tackle box each day, promising to hook us a barramundi for tea, but try as he might, the mighty fish eluded him. Eventually, the old digger who owned the caravan park took pity on him and shared the location to his secret fishing spot, claiming it was home to some of the biggest barra in the area. He drew us a map on the back of a napkin, marking the spot with an X, and that afternoon we set off.

As darkness descended, we reached the secret location; a large, swampy billabong surrounded by tall reeds. A battered old boat, a 'tinny' in Aussie speak, was next to a tree where a gap led down to the water. We pushed the tinny to the water's edge. It was pitch black apart from our torchlight. From somewhere in the darkness I heard a strange rumbling that raised the hairs on the back of my neck. I wasn't the kind to back away from an adventure, but my Spidey sense was tingling big time. There was a loud splash nearby.

'Fair dinkum, those barra sound big,' whispered Trev excitedly.

'I don't think that was a fish,' I said, scanning the reeds with my torch.

'She'll be right. Hop in, and I'll push us out. When we're free of these reeds I can motor out into the clear water.'

Trev's first cast landed close to a submerged tree whose bleached branches resembled the bones of an ancient dinosaur. I was a little on edge but had unwavering faith in Trev to keep me safe. As he began winding in his lure, I shined my torch around the billabong. The shallow water near the banks lit up like a string of oversized fairy lights. Eerie yellow eyes were everywhere. Crocodiles. Big ones.

'Trev,' I whispered, 'we've got company.' I pointed my torchlight at the ripples of a very large croc coming for us.

'No worries mate. We're in a tinny, safe as houses.'

No sooner had the words left his mouth than another two crocs surfaced near the boat and began swimming in circles around us. I tried to make myself as small as I could in the centre of the little tinny.

'Trev?' I questioned, concerned.

'Yeah, I saw 'em.'

The tenor of his voice gave away the fact his confidence was wavering. He reeled in his line, put down his rod and began desperately trying to start the engine. I felt a bump as one of the crocs nudged the tinny, testing its strength. Or perhaps it was hoping one of the idiots inside would roll out. The motor finally spluttered and kicked in. Trev aimed the tinny for the gap in the reeds where we'd come from and drove it straight out of the water and onto the bank, tipping the engine so the prop was still spinning but not biting the ground. He killed the motor and we leapt out, running to the safety of the 4WD. We slammed the doors and jammed down the locks. Our hearts were hammering in our chests. I shined my torch into the blackness. Pairs of yellow eyes stared at us from the water's edge.

'Holy hell,' I laughed. 'I can't believe that just happened!'

'Ah, we were all good. I had it totally under control.'

He smiled sheepishly. 'Takeaway fish and chips for tea?'

'Crazy Aussie.'

Having survived our croc encounter, our next stop was a remote cattle station owned by Trev's brother-in-law and his family. It was literally in the middle of nowhere: half a million acres of land located a seven-hour drive southwest of Katherine over rough, dusty, unsealed roads with no speed limits. The mail was delivered by plane once a week, the closest neighbour was an hour's drive away and the nearest pub was more than 300 km away. If at any time you became seriously ill, your only chance of survival was the flying doctor, an on-call ambulance in the sky.

'This is a working cattle station, it ain't no holiday resort,' Nathan announced to us on our arrival. Nathan was Trev's brother-in-law, and he wasn't kidding. The family and staff toiled from sunup to sundown, and we were invited to join in the hard, dusty work of mustering wild cattle by horseback and helicopter. After being corralled in the yards, the calves and yearlings were separated from their mothers, branded, dehorned, ear tagged, and the males castrated. I loved every minute of it, even the castrating bit. Often, the Aboriginal stockmen and cattle dogs would joyfully chew on the 'bush oysters' after searing them on a hot plate next to the branding iron fire. They offered some to me, but I shook my head vehemently. Guess I had a ways to go before I became a real jillaroo. I was still trying to convince myself that the docile, grass-munching vegetarians we had rounded up were actually hardy, half-wild, outback survivors. My naiveté almost cost me my life. As usual, Trev had my back.

I was sitting on the rails watching the action in the yards when I heard the ringing of the homestead lunch bell. We'd been working the cattle under the blazing sun since early morning, and I was hot, hungry and thirsty. I jumped down from the wooden fence and absentmindedly crossed the cattle yards, salivating over the thought of a sizzling steak-and-onion sandwich. I saw Trev across the yard and waved. A look of intense fear flashed across his face.

'Get the hell out of there!' he yelled, pointing behind me.

I glanced over my shoulder. A huge Brahman bull was foaming at the mouth, one leg aggressively pawing the ground, eyes glaring at me with malicious intent as it prepared to charge. Without having to be told twice, I took off for the fence as fast as my little legs could carry me. Behind me, I heard and felt the pounding of hundreds of kilos of solid muscle connecting with the ground as the beast closed in. The bull was determined to teach me a lesson about who was boss of the yards. I knew the bull was close, but just how close I wasn't sure and I didn't dare look. A metre away from the fence I launched myself into the air and onto the rails where Trev was waiting. He reached down and yanked me upwards, just as the bull slammed into the railings below.

'Bloody hell, you okay?'

Trev spun me round looking for puncture wounds.

'Yep. Had it totally under control. Steak and chips for tea?'

He shook his head. 'Crazy Canadian.'

As I lay in the swag that night, I watched the embers of the campfire drift into the heavens and reminisced about the last few months. It had been a whirlwind of a journey so far, and I finally felt like I was living my dream. I'd filled the hole in my soul. For once in my life I felt like there was no more itch left to scratch. I was part of a world with no rules and raw edges, snuggled up next to the man I loved, thousands of miles away from the civilised world. It was exhilarating and wild and not everyone's cup of tea, but for someone like me who thrived living life on the edge, it was heaven. This was the adventure I'd imagined for myself when I first shined my flashlight on the icicles outside my window 20 years earlier.

I marvelled at the power of manifestation. It wasn't like I ever had any idea of how I'd get to the Land Down Under when I was a kid, yet here I was, smelling the eucalypts and the red earth, feeling connected, whole...alive. Maybe it wasn't so much about focusing on a particular object or place but on having a clear vision of a destination full of adventure in which I was content and sharing my joy with others.

It was now early December. We'd been at the station for two weeks, and Trev was keen to take me back to his farm in Jrudgerie to meet his family for Christmas. We still had a 9,000-kilometre journey ahead of us through the states of Western Australia, South Australia and New South Wales. It was going to be a very long road trip. The entire station turned out to see us off. As we waved goodbye Trev inserted a cassette and cranked up 'Slice of Heaven' by Dave Dobbyn and the Herbs. We hit the red earth highway singing madly along to the chorus, our love shining over the horizon as we revelled in our own little slice of heaven.

Over the next week, we drove for countless hours on endless stretches of road linking Broome to Perth and Bunbury to Broken Hill. We made a sightseeing stop to watch one of the world's most stunning sunsets at beautiful Cable Beach near Broome. Then it was on to the legendary Nullarbor Plain, a 1200-kilometre expanse of flat, scrubby bush that stretched from Norseman in Western Australia all the way to Ceduna in South Australia. Summer had arrived with a vengeance and the temperature was pushing over 40°C.

I certainly couldn't complain about getting my share of the blistering hot Aussie sun. The long hours in the 4WD gave Trevor plenty of time to fill me in on his life in Jrudgerie and provide an in-depth description of everything wonderful about his town and family.

'Jrudgerie may be small, but fair dinkum, I love the place. Everyone knows everyone, and we all look out for each other.'

He described the family farm, which grew fat, golden heads of wheat in winter, paddocks of lush, green rice in the summer and tomatoes so sweet you could eat them like apples. I was entranced. He made it sound like Utopia. He told me about his loving mother, an amazing cook who was adored by the whole town, and about his father, his best mate.

'Dad's gonna love you. He's a great bloke. Before I went travelling, we worked a lot together, sometimes on the farm, but mostly painting houses, and often my Pop worked alongside us too. Three generations swingin' a brush.'

He spun me stories of an idyllic childhood growing up with his three gorgeous sisters. He spoke lovingly of his grandfather, the life and soul of every party, who had recently bought an old 'fixer-upper' cottage in town. Trev planned to help him renovate it when we got back.

Trev's stories excited me. I couldn't wait to meet these wonderful people, especially after being away from my own family for so long. While I was a little sad our road trip was ending, I was looking forward to the next exciting chapter of my life with my 'naked surfer dude'. Finally, after passing through Broken Hill and several other outback New South Wales towns, we reached the sign we'd been waiting to see for 9,000 long kilometres: *Welcome to Jrudgerie Shire*. I looked expectantly at Trevor. Surely, any minute now, we would enter the oasis of green and gold he'd rhapsodised about with so much passion. But instead, all I could see around me were flat, brown fields covered in tumbleweed and a muddy, man-made lake. Was this the sparkling body of water he skied on every summer? Confusion hit me as we pulled onto the main street. Surely this couldn't be it? Jrudgerie was desolate, dreary and depressing. It literally hurt my eyes.

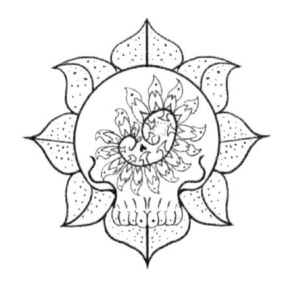

CHAPTER EIGHTEEN
The Sleeping Dragon Awakes

People don't fear change, they fear the loss that change brings.
~ Don Carmont

Jrudgerie, centre of the known universe, or at least Trevor's anyway. Total population approximately 800 true blue Aussie souls. One main street, four pubs, a bowling club, a golf club and a 'gourmet' Chinese restaurant for those special occasion dinners. Okay, so the town wasn't particularly ugly or hellish, it just lacked charm and charisma and was typical of most small outback settlements; surrounded as it was by very flat, very boring, very dry farmland. As a Canadian used to Toronto's multicultural shopping precincts and a countryside characterised by rolling green hills and snow-covered pine forests, I found the drought-stricken landscape harsh and depressing. Its only saving grace seemed to be the occasional swathe of brilliant green rice paddies and food crops fed by the giant Murray–Darling river system, the sole reason for Jrudgerie's continued existence.

In stark contrast to the town's unappealing nature, Trevor's family was beautiful, inside and out. His dad was old school, a hard worker with street smarts and a heart of gold. By day he painted, and at night and on the weekends he farmed. Trev's mum was an angel, a treasure, a ton of fun, exactly as Trev had described, and I loved her from the day we met. We spent nights on the veranda of the family farmhouse, sipping champagne and talking about anything and everything while surrounded by the vast, starry skies.

As for Trev's three sisters, what can I say? They were stunning, with golden, glossy hair, blue eyes and perfectly aerobicised bodies. They looked incredible in everything they wore, as if they'd leapt off the cover of *Vogue*. I found it hard to believe they'd grown up in Jrudgerie. They were the complete antithesis to Trevor's shirtless, shoeless, country hick demeanour. I felt inadequate around them in my well-worn backpacker duds and hair that had only recently been cut and styled by their brother. Initially, I thought girls this perfect would have to be either bimbos or bitches, but they were quick-witted and warm-hearted. It was they who taught me to become an aerobics instructor and instilled in me a lifelong passion for teaching fitness. I wasn't sure who I loved more, Trevor or his family.

When Christmas Day finally rolled around it was hot as hell and dry as a bone, yet I found myself enjoying life at the family farm. There was a certain kind of beauty that paralleled the harshness, even though it sure didn't feel like the Christmas holidays without snow. Sadly, the festive occasion was marred by Trev's grandad dying of a heart attack while teeing off from the 16th hole, just two days before Christmas. He was something of a legend, and the whole town mourned for him. Trev in particular was devastated. They'd been very close.

Following the funeral and the tick-over of the New Year, I began counting down the days until my departure. My visa expired in March, and Trev and I planned on returning to Canada. In the meantime, to keep busy and earn some money, I helped the family in their painting business and weeded row upon endless row of tomatoes. Trevor had never been overseas—well, not unless you counted Tasmania—and was super excited about the trip. I was too, but for different reasons. Jrudgerie had turned out to be achingly boring. It was one thing travelling and having adventures in the remote outback, quite another spending my days watching paint dry and pulling weeds on semi-arid plains. Even our Friday night excitement was lame. It consisted mostly of buying tickets for the meat raffle and playing the hand-cranked pokies at the local golf club. At one point Trev's sister asked me if I thought I'd ever return to Jrudgerie to live.

'Not a chance,' I replied emphatically.

Two long months passed before it was finally time to leave. I was busting for Trev to meet all my family back in Canada. I was also keen to show Trev all my favourite Bali spots and for him to experience the culture. Then there was my wild gin and tonic-loving Aunt Kath and the family in California, not to mention some surfing in Hawaii. Suffice to say, over the next month of our overseas travel, we had a blast at every single one of our holiday destinations, especially with Aunt Kath, before finally making it to my home town of Toronto.

As I expected, my entire family fell in love with Trev. Not surprisingly, they had no clue where Jrudgerie actually was. 'Four hours north of Melbourne' only elicited shakes of the head. Trev patiently explained where he lived and waxed lyrical about the beauty of his town while I sat in the background, rolling my eyes.

Dad found Trev's passion for everything, including the mundane, highly amusing. But he was over the moon when he found out he had both a keen golfer and handyman living under his roof. Trev's handyman skills were forever in demand, not only by my labour-averse Dad but also by the entire neighbourhood. Trev had done the rounds on the golf course and introduced himself to everyone who lived within three city blocks.

It didn't take long before everyone had heard of 'Trevor Donovan from Jrudgerie'. He was never a day without work. I was thrilled to have my job back at the gym, but despite over a year having passed, I was still the butt of many a joke thanks to my purchase of a member for an exorbitant sum of money at the MS charity auction. Buddha once said happiness is wanting nothing more than what you have at the moment, and that pretty much summed up my life during this time. I had it all. I was home with my wonderful family, I had a job I enjoyed and a man I loved. My existence was bliss. But then something strange happened.

I awoke one morning with a searing pain in my right shoulder. I tried to remember what I'd done to aggravate it. Perhaps it was because I repeatedly pushed myself hard at the gym—'No pain, no gain' was the motto I lived by—but this seemed to be different. It felt more like a pinched nerve rather than anything muscular, and even after several weeks it hadn't subsided. The final indignity came when the weakness and pain in my right arm pushed me off the squash competition leaderboard. I was told politely it might be best if I hung up my racquet for the season.

I went to doctors, had X-rays, saw chiropractors and massage therapists. Nobody seemed to have an answer, but everyone had a theory. Damaged nerve, soft tissue injury, carpal tunnel, frozen shoulder—nobody could pinpoint the problem. I ate anti-inflammatories for breakfast, lunch and dinner. Eventually, however, I lost the use of my right arm and hand altogether. I couldn't hold a pen or guide a fork to my mouth. I had no control and zero sensation from my shoulder down, no understanding of where my arm was in space unless I was actually looking at it.

One night while out for dinner with a friend, we smelled something burning. It was my hand. It had been perched over a burning candle for so long that my cuff had started to smoulder and my skin had started to blister. My friend grabbed my arm and poured water over it. My cuff was blackened and my hand burnt, but there was no feeling, no sensation of pain. It was strange and scary.

Now I'm not the sort to wallow in self-pity—in fact, I try to make light of any bad situation. I believe in accepting what is and moving on, like a river flowing around a rock. But it's never easy practising acceptance when you've lost the use of a precious limb. At this stage I had no idea whether my loss was temporary or permanent. It was all new territory for me. What I did know however, was that fighting change was a prescription for suffering. I needed to accept the loss of movement and function of my right arm and instead focus on trying to improve the functionality of my left. I'd already learned to live with a temporary handicap after being hit by a motorbike in Bali, so this wasn't a mental stretch for me. Plus, I could tolerate pain thanks to the migraines of my early years and my time in the army. No, this was about convincing myself that everything would be okay.

I did my best to remain positive, but being a one-armed lefty created major challenges for me. Before widespread computer use, my job as a salesperson entailed writing out contracts. My handwriting has been described as atrocious at the best of times. Now my manager likened my left-handed penmanship to the scribblings of a serial killer. I also hadn't realised how handy it was to have two arms to put on knickers or jeans. I felt like I was constantly losing at a game of Twister.

Trev, in the meantime, had been on 'walkabout' around western Canada. When he returned, I didn't want to worry him with my arm issues so I played down the problem and my ever-increasing challenges. His visa was about to expire, and although he was sad about leaving, I knew he was looking forward to going back to the wide-open, flat, boring nothingness of Jrudgerie. How anyone could miss that place was beyond my comprehension. It was a heartbreaking, tearful farewell at the airport, neither of us sure what would happen next. We were from opposite ends of the planet and from very different worlds.

Whoever coined the term 'lovesick' nailed it. Physical pain is one thing, emotional pain a whole different kettle of fish. Over the next two weeks Trev and I made long, expensive calls every few days to each other, and each time we hung up, all I longed to do was talk to him again. When I couldn't take it anymore, I caved and bought a ticket back to Oz. Dad wasn't surprised.

'What took you so long? He's been gone an entire 14 days.'

'I know, right?! But two more sleeps and I'm outta here, flying over that great big, blue ocean. I'm just not sure how I'm going to handle 20 hours on a plane with this bloody painful shoulder.'

My dad, the banker, was a man who relied on hard facts to make important decisions, so I was pretty surprised when he suggested I give acupuncture a shot.

'Well, you've tried everything else,' he said logically. 'What's there to lose? No worse than those pills you keep popping.'

So that afternoon I found myself in the little Chinese clinic right next to the shop where, five years earlier, I'd met Glenn the coupon salesman while chewing on a Twizzler. Acupuncture. Even the name filled me with dread. I still hated needles with a passion, but I was desperate and had promised Dad to give it a go. An old, bespectacled Chinese lady smelling faintly of soy sauce and fried chicken began flicking needles into my head. I felt like I was going to vomit and faint at the same time. She ignored my grimaces and sickly pallor and began twisting the needles into my flesh, smiling and nodding like a mad, mediaeval torturer. I swear she enjoyed the experience as much as I hated it. I was so traumatised afterwards, I couldn't even stomach a Twizzler, but when I got home and Dad asked how I felt, I realised the pain had gone. For now, at least, the victory went to Chinese medicine, and I put away the ibuprofen.

A day later I boarded the plane to Oz and, after 20 hours of pain-free travel, found myself being greeted at Melbourne airport by my Aussie surfer dude, who lived nowhere near the ocean, proudly holding a sign saying: *Trevor Donovan from Jrudgerie*. I melted.

I knew this reunion meant living in his little outback town, miles from anywhere, a place I'd sworn ten months earlier I'd never return to on a full-time basis, but love trumps all. And so I settled into a life of drudgery in Jrudgerie and resigned myself to my destiny, in this case helping Trev with his painting. It soon became apparent, however, that even though the acupuncture had taken my pain away, it hadn't restored the function of my arm. At the insistence of Trev's mum I went to see yet another doctor who referred me to a neurologist in Melbourne. Thank God for concerned mothers. The referral turned out to be my salvation.

The neurologist's name was so long he encouraged me to simply call him Dr Alphabet. He was of Indian descent and had intelligent brown eyes, a cultured English accent and a calm, caring demeanour. He was sympathetic when I explained how disappointed I was about my defunct squash game.

'Let's see what's going on. Close your eyes. Now touch your right index finger to your nose.'

I failed miserably.

'Okay,' he said encouragingly, 'Now open them, and try again.'

With my eyes wide open, I tried again but it still didn't work. He put a pencil in my hand, palm faced down, and wrapped my fingers around it. The pencil immediately fell to the floor, which did not surprise me. It did not seem to surprise him either.

'One last thing. Try to touch your thumb to each of your fingers.'

I almost laughed at the absurdity of the request. 'Sorry. You might as well ask me to levitate!'

I felt like a failure. Dr Alphabet nodded, then reached for the phone.

'I want to send you for a few more tests, Kat. An MRI and then a lumbar puncture.'

I was horrified. The doctor who I'd thought so kind and gentle was now asking me to endure a procedure that was my worst nightmare: a bloody big needle stuck directly into my spine.

A few days later I was called back to the office, still slightly traumatised after the lumbar puncture episode. Dr Alphabet explained the MRI had shown inflammation in a part of my brain responsible for the movement of my arm. The tests revealed an elevated white blood cell count. There could be a number of reasons for this, he said, but for now he suggested four days' worth of intravenous methylprednisolone, a steroid. Really? Four months of suffering with a paralysed arm, and I could be cured with a drug bodybuilders took to grow bigger muscles?

The irony of the situation wasn't lost on me. I'd spent most of my time in Canada working and training at a gym full of 'roid-fuelled bodybuilders. I checked into St Vincent's hospital and within 48 hours I could miraculously touch my finger to my thumb. On day four I even managed to sign my discharge papers from the hospital with my right hand. Disaster averted. I was cured!

Sadly, the same positive outcome didn't hold true for my Jrudgerie experience. The euphoric high of my rejuvenated arm was soon replaced by the soul-depleting low of living in the ass-end of nowhere doing jobs I disliked. Being in Jrudgerie with the man I loved was proving to be a double-edged sword. On the one hand, I was no longer lovesick and I was able to spend time with Trevor's beautiful family. On the other, I was once again stuck living in Hicksville. To make matters worse, we'd moved from the family farm into town so Trev could finish renovating the dilapidated cottage he'd bought from his grandfather's estate. We'd morphed into a new subspecies: country townies.

The cottage was right on the main highway. Semi-trailers roared by day and night, causing the windows to rattle and the fresh country air to become tainted with the aroma and carcinogens of diesel fumes. I'd gone from falling in love with Trev surrounded by the heavenly turquoise waters of Airlie Beach to living with him on a highway to hell.

We often discussed moving out of Jrudgerie once the cottage was finished, perhaps to a place near the ocean in Queensland, but we didn't set a timeline and the house renovations were never-ending. Life became a series of overlapping, repeating events—painting, sanding, cleaning, weeding—topped off by pots of beer and meat raffles at the golf club on a Friday night. Groundhog Day, Jrudgerie style!

I was fast reaching breaking point. Soon, I'd have to face a heart-wrenching decision, to either stay with the man I believed was my destiny or leave to reclaim my spark for life, my sense of self and my passion for adventure.

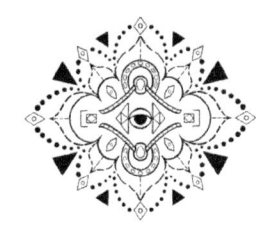

CHAPTER NINETEEN
Fake It 'Til You Make It

Train yourself to let go of everything you fear to lose.
- Yoda

Life in Jrudgerie affected me in a hundred small ways. I became irritated, frustrated, bored and I once again felt I had an itch I couldn't scratch. I found myself taking out my frustrations on Trev. He responded by retreating into his man cave, the shed out the back, and doing whatever the hell it is men do in there. This, of course, led me to become even more irritated.

I had no real friends of my own, unless you counted Ethel, the dear old lady across the road. My closest confidants were Trev's sisters and his mum, which made things awkward as I found myself unloading, in less than favourable terms, about the son and brother they loved. To their credit, they did their best to support me, but the gnawing emptiness inside me grew like a weed and the endless expanse of wide-open spaces around me only seemed to magnify my inner landscape of loneliness and isolation. It was no surprise when the gloss started wearing off our fairytale romance. As much as Trevor and I had a deep love for each other, we also on occasion had an equally deep dislike for each other. We began to argue...a lot. The honeymoon was over.

I called an old friend, Sandra, for advice. I first met Sandra in Toronto when we were eight years old. We bonded during Sunday school while in detention in the hallway, mostly on account of me talking to her during class. She was now working in Rome as an English teacher but was about to move to Tuscany to work at an elite summer camp in the mountains. When she heard of my troubles she suggested I join her, saying she could wrangle me a job there as an English teacher. A summer in the mountains of Tuscany certainly sounded like a much better option than spending a chilly winter in the dreary outback. I didn't need any more convincing.

I bought a ticket, packed my bag, and a few weeks later it was time to go. Trev and I were unsure where our future lay. We loved one another, but was that enough? At the airport we were both emotional, neither of us knowing whether this would be a forever goodbye. I promised Trev I'd keep in touch, which in the pre-Facebook late 90s, meant snail mail and dumping a truckload of coins into a payphone. On the plane to Italy, I agonised over my decision to leave. Part of me hoped our love would be like a boomerang, one you could throw with blind faith deep into the wilderness, confident it would come back.

But even if it did, I wasn't sure if our relationship was strong enough to withstand the monotony of life in an isolated country town. Perhaps by leaving I could put my theory to the test and discover once and for all whether or not we were really meant to be together. Either way, wanderlust had seduced me with the promise of an adventure in Tuscany.

Sandra greeted me in Rome dressed in running gear. Although I'd been awake for three days travelling on planes, trains and automobiles, I agreed that running around a hot and humid city was indeed the perfect way to overcome jet lag. We dropped my backpack at her Uncle Mario's apartment and set off. I poured my heart out as we jogged past the Colosseum, the Vatican and dozens of other iconic Italian landmarks. Sandra doled out some much-needed support, then gave me a rundown of my new job, including the fact she may have led the camp director to believe my English teaching experience was more extensive than it actually was, which was zero. In other words, I was about to be gainfully employed in a job for which I was grossly ill-equipped. But far from stressing out about the idea, I decided I would relish the challenge and vowed to dive into my new role as a 'maestra' with passion and commitment.

It wasn't in my nature to allow a lack of education or know-how to stand in my way of doing anything. Then again, this wasn't the first time in my life I'd adopted the Fake It 'Till You Make It strategy, which my grandfather, Papa Joe, had taught me. I'd used it on many different occasions to gain illegal entry into bars, apply for jobs well above my skill level and push through physical challenges I wasn't quite conditioned for. Whenever my self-confidence wavered and I needed to convince myself I was better or stronger than I was, I'd tell myself, 'Come on girl, fake it 'til you make it!'

It was only later in life that I discovered science actually backed me up. Essentially, pumping up self-belief acts like a placebo effect for the soul. Forcing a smile even when you're not happy, for example, can trick your brain into believing you're happy, which then triggers a release of dopamine and serotonin to spur actual happiness. My use of this strategy has, over the years, allowed me to become comfortable with discomfort, suffer fewer regrets and live fearlessly outside my comfort zone while reducing anxiety and stress. It's led to a profound shift in how I approach challenges. So, for me, swallowing a little pill of self-belief seemed like the ideal solution to overcoming my shortcomings of being responsible for the education of a bunch of Italian kids.

The route to the camp, located at the top of a majestic mountain in the Lucca countryside, passed through a beautiful valley lined with ancient vineyards and olive and chestnut groves. It also skirted a number of historic walled villages. This was a world far removed from Jrudgerie. 'Camp' was actually a bit of a misnomer for the facility. Rather than canvas tents, staff and students were housed in beautiful, old stone buildings with red-tiled roofs and white-rendered walls. This was a summer school for kids of the rich and famous. Their parents generally stayed at the luxurious five-star hotel at the base of the mountain. The school's director—a slender, slightly effeminate Englishman—proved to be kind and generous and seemed not to notice my shortcomings as a teacher, or perhaps he liked me well enough to politely ignore them.

English was never my strongest subject and, embarrassingly, some of the students in my class could spell better than me. Thanks to lots of clandestine coaching by Sandra and a can-do attitude, I mastered the basics of teaching quite rapidly. I made up for my lack of experience with humour, passion and commitment, teaching English in my own, idiosyncratic way. Often this involved hauling my students outside and making them do exercises while yelling out English phrases.

When not teaching, I ran the mountain trails. It was heaven. This place was everything Jrudgerie was not: vivid greens, colourful wildflowers, bubbling streams cascading through picturesque valleys and ravines. There were endless adventures to be had and, of course, exquisite Italian food and wine to indulge in. The ten of us employed as English teachers hailed from all over the world, including England, America, Holland, Germany, and Switzerland. I was the only one who didn't speak fluent Italian, and I was determined to learn.

Whenever we went into the nearby village, a half-hour walk down the mountain, I would ask my friends to teach me how to order our food in Italian. This often opened up all sorts of doors for hilarity at my expense. While imbibing at a local trattoria one evening, instead of ordering three glasses of white wine and a platter of meat, my friends had me asking for three extra-large condoms and a man with a large penis. The bartender shook his hands in the air and yelled, 'Cosa? Mama mia, non qui!' Which roughly translated to, 'What the? Oh my God, not here!'

Despite these many embarrassing situations, or perhaps because of them, I quickly picked up the language. After a few months, both my Italian and my teaching techniques had improved immensely, but by then my summer job in the mountains of Tuscany was coming to an end. A group of us, including Sandra, Richard from Britain and Christian from Switzerland, made plans to head off on an extended European road trip. I had no idea this would prove to be a pivotal moment in my life and help unearth my mother's fascinating history and heritage. Its effect on me would be profound.

CHAPTER TWENTY
A Taste of the Past

*Nikdy nemůžete přeplout oceán, dokud nebudete mít
odvahu ztratit břeh z očí.*
You can never cross the ocean until you have the
courage to lose sight of the shore.
~ Czech proverb

Christian crouched low and shuffled gingerly across the narrow ice bridge spanning the crevasse. We'd overwhelmingly nominated him as the sacrificial lamb of our tiny teacher flock. Not just because he was the oldest and most experienced climber among us but also because he was the biggest and we figured if he didn't break through the ice and die, then none of us would either. He stepped as lightly as he could from one narrow ledge to the next. Some of the ice bridges were less than two metres wide. We held our collective breath as we watched him. All around us the ice creaked and moaned incessantly. There was a loud crack as a large chunk fell away from underneath him into the dark recesses of the abyss below. We waited for the sound of it to hit bottom. It was a long time coming. Christian froze in his tracks. He carefully checked the ice around him for any telltale signs of cracks then gave us the okay signal. Phew! We watched as he inched slowly forwards. After what seemed like an eternity, he stepped across the other side to safety. Now it was my turn.

I made a mental note of where Christian had traversed and did my best to follow his footprints in the snow. I shuffled out onto the ice, crouching as low as possible, imitating Christian's stance. The light covering of snow provided some grip, but anywhere there was bare ice proved to be dangerously slippery. I was wearing my favourite, well-worn blue runners, not exactly ideal for ice climbing, but I felt they provided me with a modicum of good luck. As I concentrated on putting one foot in front of the other and testing the ice for strength, Christian doled out encouragement and instructions to me from the safety of the other side. I studiously avoided looking into the abyss below, heeding Dad's advice from back when he taught me to drive: *'If you don't want to drive into a tree—don't look at it.'*

This time there was no loud crack, just an ominous creaking. I didn't know which was worse. I consoled myself with the mantra that if it was my time to die, it was my time to die and that at least I would go out doing something adventurous rather than sanding door frames in Jrudgerie. Strangely, I also found myself wishing I could see Trev again. My love for him, it seemed, still burned strong somewhere deep inside of me and wouldn't let me go. And then suddenly I felt Christian's hand grip my arm and yank me off the ice and onto solid rock. I'd made it! Guess it wasn't my time to die after all.

I took time out to reflect on the moment. It was mostly my fault we'd been placed in this predicament, a result of my insatiable appetite for adventure and my predilection not to play by the rules. Our hike had started off easy enough, a four-hour, non-technical climb to the top of a small mountain peak in Switzerland. However, when we reached the top, I suggested looking for another way down, one that was more challenging, despite a sign warning us in four different languages not to stray off the designated path. Surprisingly, everyone agreed except for Sandra, who was perpetually risk averse. But eventually, I convinced even her to come with us, pointing out it was a perfect day and that going down would be far easier and faster than going up. What could possibly go wrong?

In the end, we all survived the 'Kat'astrophe of the crevasse. We celebrated with a bottle of wine and a never-to-be-forgotten Swiss fondue in an alpine hut at the base of the mountain later that night. After dinner, Sandra launched into an 'I told you so' speech, ending with, 'Seriously girl, you are always getting me into trouble!'

I countered with, 'But it was a fun adventure, right?'

She groaned in frustration. 'We nearly died! Weren't you scared?'

'Yep, but I loved every minute of it.'

And it was true, I wasn't afraid of dying, although Sandra did have a point. Maybe we should have stuck to the well-worn path. Unfortunately, I was an unapologetic risk-taker who thrived on adrenaline and viewed any obstacle placed in front of me as a challenge to be overcome, even if it meant inadvertently putting others in harm's way. I wasn't quite sure where this came from. It was as if I was born with a 'never say die' attitude hard-wired into my DNA.

The rest of our European holiday wasn't quite as dramatic as our alpine adventure, but we still had some wild times. We drove through the south of France and kayaked down the Ardèche. We camped at Cannes and hung out at Monaco's bars and beaches. And then we wound our way back up the northern mountains of Italy to the city of Trento so Sandra and Christian could compete in a field hockey tournament.

Although I was missing Trev, I had no intention of returning to Jrudgerie anytime soon. He was still renovating the cottage, and I was thoroughly enjoying my European adventures. But something else was nagging me, something I couldn't quite put my finger on. And then it came to me. Despite having been immersed in Italian, Swiss and French culture and having European blood coursing through my veins, I still felt like I didn't truly 'belong' to any of the countries I'd visited. Yes, I found them exciting, stimulating, fascinating, but nothing felt 'familiar', nothing triggered my childhood memories or meshed with my family's stories—at least the ones instilled into me by my mother and grandmother.

Then fate intervened in the form of a Czech men's hockey team. I heard their name being announced as winners of their division while cheering on Sandra and Richard from the sidelines. Holy moly, this had to be a sign! Mum had always wanted to take us kids back to Czechoslovakia but she was unable to because, as a defector, she would have been arrested and jailed if she returned. The Iron Curtain didn't fall until five years after she'd died. Now here at last was a chance to fulfil my mother's wishes.

The team wasn't hard to find with their newly presented medals draped around their necks. I strode up and asked if I could hitch a ride with them to the Czech Republic but none of them understood English. It took a lot of miming, pointing to myself and then to the bus, to explain what I wanted to do. Confusion reigned until a player who spoke English arrived. His name was Matyas, and he translated my request to their coach. What followed was no doubt an animated discussion as to who the hell this crazy girl was and why she wanted to hitch a ride, but in the end they unanimously and graciously agreed I could be a stowaway. I was elated. I chose to see this as vindication of my impetuousness, a sliding-door moment that would finally enable me to connect with my roots. I ran to grab my belongings from Christian's Pinto, then made a quick collect call to my grandmother in Canada. My Nana expressed concern about my trip and wondered who would do such a thing with zero forward planning. Eventually, she stopped lecturing me long enough to give me some contact names and numbers.

My travelling companions didn't seem at all surprised I was off on another wild adventure. Sandra shook her head, enveloped me in a big bear hug and wished me luck. And just like that I was off, travelling on a bus to God knows where in the

Czech Republic with an 18-member, all-male field hockey team. Crazy? Possibly. Bordering on madness? Maybe. But the risks never crossed my mind because I was finally on my way to my mother's homeland.

I bumped along in the bus, surrounded by sweaty boys. As Belgium whipped by in the dark, I co-opted Matyas to teach me some rudimentary Czech. I knew I wouldn't get far saying only 'ahoj' to everyone. I learned a few handy words and phrases, like 'Dobre rano', which meant good morning. Somewhere in the deepest dark of night, the bus pulled into a rural town. I had no idea where I was or where I would stay. When my new friend Matyas offered me a couch at his parents' home, I gratefully accepted. The next morning, his poor mother, dressed in a housecoat and with rollers in her hair, was shocked to find a strange girl sleeping on her sofa.

'Ahoj, dobre rano, me Kat,' I ventured, patting myself on the chest and feeling very uncomfortable.

It was an awkward few hours waiting for Matyas to wake up and explain who I was.

My grandmother had made arrangements for me to stay with her oldest friend, Otto, and later that day Matyas drove me to the city of Brno to meet him. Otto greeted me like a long-lost family member. He had a tear in his eye as he remarked how much I looked like my grandmother when she was my age. He'd already planned all the places he wanted to show me, including where my mother was born. Otto's tiny apartment was in a drab grey residential block of classically Communist-era design. He was a gentle soul, in his mid-seventies, tall, distinguished, with thinning hair and a neatly trimmed grey beard and moustache. He spoke just enough English for us to communicate. Olga, his shorter, stockier, apron-clad wife, spoke no English at all, so she and I bonded over the universal language of food.

When I arrived Olga just happened to be preparing one of my favourite childhood dishes, knedliky, a carb and fat-laden meal I used to help Mum make. It was classic Czech cuisine, consisting of a dough made from mashed potatoes and flour. We broke off bits of the dough, rolled them into balls and stuffed them with chunks of sweet, juicy, ripe plums, then dropped them into boiling water. When they were ready, they floated to the top where we scooped them out. Just before serving them we drowned the dumplings in salty melted butter, sprinkled them with poppy seeds and dusted them with icing sugar—sweet, salty, savoury, all packed into one scrumptious mouthful. As soon as I tasted one I was transported back in time to my mother's kitchen. I closed my eyes and sighed. I'd found the connection I'd been seeking. I was home.

When Otto asked if I was ready to see where my mother grew up, I vigorously nodded my head. I'd been waiting my whole life for this. It was like being given a magic key to Mum's memories and childhood, things she rarely talked about because it always seemed to make her sad. Otto drove me past row upon row of identical grey apartment blocks until we reached a more elaborate, Baroque-style building in the centre of the city. We climbed three flights of stairs to the top floor, hoping we'd be allowed to look inside the apartment. When we knocked on the door, a heavy-set lady with grey hair pulled back into a severe bun answered almost immediately. Otto explained why we were there, and she warmly invited us in.

The first thing I noticed was the sweet, savoury smell of frying onions and that immediately reminded me of my mum again. I was amazed at how bright and airy the apartment was. It had high ceilings finished with detailed mouldings. There were three bedrooms, a large living room and a decent-sized kitchen. This was not like Otto's dreary apartment at all. As we looked out one of the big crossbar windows onto the street below, I had a flashback to when I was little: Mum telling me how her family shared this apartment with another couple and how they'd stood in line for hours in the freezing cold outside the butcher shop in the street below because food was so scarce.

'Your mum was 17 when she left here,' commented Otto, interrupting my thoughts. 'Your grandparents sent her to live with cousins in America to escape the Communist regime.'

The plan had been to get everyone out, but they couldn't all leave together without raising suspicion. My determined grandmother never gave up trying to escape. However, it was not until four years later, when the Russians invaded Prague in the spring of '68, that she got her chance.

'The troops marched right past this window,' Otto gestured to the street below, as if he could still see the invading forces. 'Your uncle was a teenager. He and his friends ran around removing street signs to mislead the soldiers who were searching for dissidents.'

In the resulting confusion, my uncle escaped to Germany and my grandparents managed to sneak across the border into Austria. They had nothing but the clothes on their backs and some cash in their pockets. The family eventually reunited and immigrated to Canada.

It hit me how lucky I was to be visiting Otto of my own free will. I had a life of liberty, whereas my mum's family had lived in constant fear of the authorities, always worrying their so-called friends and neighbours would turn them in for being 'subversive'. I couldn't fathom what it must have been like for them to leave behind everything and everyone they loved and move to another country they knew little to nothing about. They'd gone with their gut instinct, making a crucial decision during a pivotal moment in their lives, staking a belief in themselves against an uncertain future in a foreign country thousands of kilometres away. Luckily, it turned out to be the right decision. Czechoslovakia spent the next 20 years under the yoke of Communism.

It occurred to me that perhaps my aversion to authority and my propensity for risk-taking behaviour was linked to this very same gut instinct, a built-in, inherited survival mechanism designed to kick in during hard times. I felt vindicated by my spontaneous decision to jump on a bus full of hockey players. I'd not only unearthed my family history and connected with Mum's heritage, but I'd also discovered my grandparents' own sliding-door moment when they seized a small window of opportunity to escape Communism. I felt strongly I was destined to be here.

'You know, this was not the first time your grandmother was involved in a dangerous escape,' Otto added.

I asked him what he meant, but he refused to elaborate.

'You need to ask her about that,' he said quietly, running a hand over his balding scalp and revealing a distinct tattoo above the wrist on his left arm.

Damn, what the hell was he talking about? What was my grandmother hiding? As far as I knew, we had no family secrets. Or did we?

I left the Czech Republic a few days later. It was time to go back to Toronto and confront my Nana about our family history.

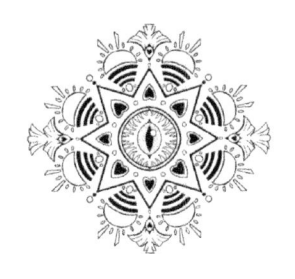

CHAPTER TWENTY-ONE
Surviving the Shoah

*When we are no longer able to change a situation,
we are challenged to change ourselves.
~ Viktor Frankl*

Growing up, I knew my mum's side of the family had arrived in Canada as refugees fleeing a life of Communism under Russian rule, but that was pretty much *all* I knew. Neither Mum nor my grandparents spoke much about their past. But in the space of one afternoon, what I thought I knew about my family history was blown apart when my Nana revealed she'd narrowly escaped death—not once but several times—at the hands of the Nazis.

For most of my life, I accepted my Czech Nana as a tough, savvy, assertive and highly capable woman who didn't stand for any crap. I never knew her to practise or subscribe to a particular religion, unlike my Dad's parents who had crosses with Jesus nailed on them hanging on every wall in their house. Looking back, however, there were a few clues. When I was ten and my grandfather died, Nana covered all the mirrors in the house with black cloth. After the funeral, my sister and I helped set the table for the wake. A man with strange hair and a little black hat scolded us for putting ham on the same table as milk. We thought it kind of odd at the time but never questioned it.

When I finally arrived on Nana's doorstep, demanding to know the truth about her life, she was taken aback.

'What exactly has Otto been telling you?'

'Nothing really. He said to ask you, but I saw his tattoo. I know what it means.' I held my breath. 'Nana?'

My grandmother stared at me for a long moment. It was clear I wasn't going to be fobbed off easily. We were very much alike in that regard.

'Okay,' she finally sighed. 'First I feed you, then we talk.'

She hauled me into the kitchen, where she proceeded to pile enough homemade cakes to feed 20 people onto a plate, then clasped my hand in hers and led me to the couch. A mixture of resignation and relief washed over her face as she began to tell her story in her thick, Slavic accent.

'My dear Katrinco, so many horrific things happened when I was young. The only way for me to live after it was all over was to keep the door closed on my memories. But you're right, this is part of who you are. You need to know.'

My grandmother was someone I'd known my whole life. But now it seemed I needed to prepare myself for the fact that maybe I'd never really known her at all. I took a deep breath and waited for her to begin.

'I was born in 1925 in Zvolen, in the Slovak region of Czechoslovakia. My brother showed up eight years later. I loved school, was top of my class, and on the weekends I rode my horse at my grandparents' farm. Our family owned a big store, it was very successful. Life was good.'

Nana's gaze was unfocused, distant, as if she were looking back through time. She continued, saying that her world changed dramatically in 1938.

'I was 13 when the government started making new rules for the Jews in Slovakia. They even passed the 'Jewish Code' a few years later in 1941—the strictest anti-Jewish laws in all of Europe. Then *pssscht*, no more school for us. We couldn't go here or there, it was like we were no longer human beings. Terrible, terrible times, Katrinco.'

I realised my Nana was confirming something I'd been wondering for a long time but never had the wherewithal to ask. My mother's family were not just immigrants from Europe but Jews who somehow survived the Holocaust. She held my hand as she patiently explained why I'd been brought up as Christian and completely missed out on my Jewish heritage.

'After the war I renounced my faith. I suffered through so many horrible atrocities and heard about so many more that I refused to believe in a God who would allow such terrible things to happen. But that doesn't mean you're not Jewish. According to Judaism, any child born to a Jewish mother is considered Jewish. But, because we stopped practising the faith, your mother was happy for your father to bring you up as a Catholic.'

193

I was Jewish? Instead of boring old Sunday school, I could've gone to bat mitzvah parties and immigrated to Israel and lived on hummus and arak and orange juice? I was stunned. As Nana refilled the teacups, I ate cake and tried to process her words. I wondered if Mum would have eventually told me. Did she even know? I was hungry for the full story and nodded for Nana to continue.

'The rules for Jews in Zvolen were very strict. We couldn't go to parks or drive cars. They took our jewellery, they even took my beautiful horse away because we weren't allowed to own pets, not even a cat.'

The memory of this seemed to anger her, even after so many years.

'We had to wear armbands with a Star of David on them so everyone would know we were Jews. Neighbours who were our friends suddenly began treating us like dirt. My father had to apply for a permit to work in his own store. Can you imagine? Another man ordered him around and took the money from his own business. Terrible!'

She ran a hand through her stylishly cropped, dyed blonde hair as if trying to calm the intensity of the memories. Nana was fighting hard to hold back tears. It was heartbreaking to see her struggling to maintain composure. I asked if she wanted to stop. She shook her head. She did her best to describe what happened next without her emotions overwhelming her. How her own country betrayed her by negotiating with the Germans to deport all Jews out of Slovakia, and how the government agreed to pay Nazi Germany 500 Reichsmarks per Jew for the cost of their 'resettlement' in work camps in Poland, beginning with single Jewish men and women.

'I had just turned 16 and was supposed to be on one of the first trains out but ended up with appendicitis in hospital. This was the first of my many lucky escapes. Not long after they began rounding up entire families. We found out later they were all being sent to their deaths.'

Thanks to her father's work permit, Nana's family managed to be exempted from the deportation lists published every Friday. However, those who were chosen had only four hours to pack their belongings and board the train. Four hours to pack up a lifetime of memories. Four hours to leave their entire world behind. Sure, I'd uprooted myself more than once at the drop of a hat, but I'd had the privilege of choosing to do so on my terms. My life was so far removed from the horrors inflicted upon these people that I found the idea of it incomprehensible.

'Why didn't they refuse or fight or hide?' I asked in disbelief.

'Because, Katrinco, the Nazis hid the truth well, and so our rabbis, our leaders said we should cooperate. They stated that as long as we were doing jobs to help the war effort, the Germans wouldn't harm us, and so people boarded the trains.'

Nana shut her eyes shut and tightened her grip on my hand. She whispered, 'They were wrong...so wrong.'

She looked at me with pain in her eyes. 'I tried my best to help in some way. I knew a few of the Slovak guards responsible for rounding up the Jews so I'd often slip them wine or alcohol that my family made. One Friday morning, I made sure to give them more than the usual amount of alcohol so they became drunk and careless. When they weren't looking, I managed to sneak a peek at the deportation lists to see whose names were on the list.

'I did my best to remember dozens and dozens of names. Then I ran to the fields where most of the Jews were being forced to work and yelled out the names. They knew exactly what it meant and I hoped to God they would run and escape.'

I sat in awe, trying to imagine my frail old nana as a young, strong, fearless teenager.

'Nana,' I exclaimed, 'You're a hero!'

I felt her fragile fist clench in my hand. 'No! No, I am not,' she replied forcefully.

'In our city of Zvolen alone, almost 69,000 out of the 89,000 Jews living there were murdered. Nearly all my family and friends were murdered. I only saved a few dozen. I should have done more to help but I was only young and didn't know how.'

Tears welled up in her eyes. I didn't know what to say to comfort her.

It wasn't long after this, she noted, when the time came that even her father's work permit wasn't enough to keep the family safe. They began hearing reports of Jewish massacres by Slovak and German soldiers in Poland and Russia. Tens of thousands of people were forced to dig their own graves before they were shot and murdered without mercy. Jewish people whispered the killings were a Shoah, an ancient Hebrew word meaning a path to complete and utter destruction. Her father began putting together a daring plan to escape Zvolen.

A few weeks later the plan finally came to fruition. The entire family boarded a train to Nitra, two hours away from Zvolen. Nitra was still inside Slovakia, but her father knew someone there who could obtain forged travel documents, allowing them to catch a second train to Hungary. While in hiding awaiting the papers, the Hlinka Guard arrived under cover of darkness, no doubt alerted by non-Jewish neighbours, and broke down the door, nearly beating my great-grandfather to death. They hauled everyone to the police station. Thankfully my great-grandfather had enough money to bribe the police to let his family go.

'After that, my father decided it would be safer if we split up,' my grandmother said. 'My little brother and I would leave straight away for Hungary. My parents would come later. I remember them putting us on the commuter train. It was a Friday, and next to us were dozens of cattle cars filled with Jews carrying suitcases, ready for so-called resettlement at the concentration camps. Truth be told, I was a little jealous of them—'

'Why Nana?' I asked, confused.

'Because they had suitcases filled with all their precious belongings, and Papa told us we couldn't carry anything. I discovered later, of course, that the resettled families never had time to unpack their bags. On arrival at the concentration camps, they were marched straight to the gas chambers and their bags were looted, then burned along with them.'

I held Nana's hands to stop them from trembling, but her voice remained calm as she recalled the rest of her journey that night, dredging up memories from the dark recesses of her mind.

'I was very nervous, very tense, sitting on the train alone with my little brother, knowing our papers only allowed us to travel within Slovakia. I was terrified of being caught, so we pretended to sleep to avoid attracting attention.'

Finally, after what seemed like an eternity, they crossed the border into Hungary. Then the door connecting the two carriages opened and the conductor entered. He demanded to see their tickets. Thinking fast, my grandmother told him they had fallen asleep and missed their stop, and so at the next station they were unceremoniously removed from the train and taken to a Hungarian police station.

'I pleaded with the officer in charge, telling him my uncle was a rich gentile who would pay for our release.' She smiled at the memory. 'Luckily, I was a very confident young woman. The officer said okay, but it would cost my uncle 600 crowns each.'

He took Nana to the post office to send a message to have the money wired to their captors, then went to a nearby restaurant to wait.

'I'll never forget that day for as long as I live. It was my 17th birthday. I hadn't eaten in over a day, and the small amount of food we had hidden in our pockets had been taken from us at the police station. I told the officer who was making a pig of himself eating a big bowl of goulash that I was hungry. He took pity on me and ordered a glass of lemonade.'

Once the money came through, just before sunrise, the policeman took Nana and her brother back to the border. He dumped them in neutral territory, a thin strip of land between Hungary and Slovakia, telling them, 'If you know what's good for you, you'll walk away and you won't let me set eyes on you again.'

With that, he left. Nana and her little brother were now stranded in the middle of nowhere in the cold, dark early hours of the morning. As they huddled together by the side of the road, a lone soldier appeared and threatened to shoot them. By this time, my grandmother had had enough.

She yelled, 'We are only children. If you're going to shoot us then do it, otherwise leave us alone!'

The soldier had second thoughts about carrying through with his threat to murder children and backed down.

Shortly afterwards, a farmer came by with his horse and carriage and agreed to take Nana and her brother to Budapest. They were elated to finally be on their way to the safety of the city. They fell asleep, only to be jolted awake when the carriage stopped and a gruff voice told them to hop out. Through bleary eyes they realised they were outside the same police station they'd left hours before! With the officer's dire warning still ringing in her ears, Nana fervently glanced around. It was still early morning and no one had seen them arrive. They quickly ran into a side street and disappeared, making their way slowly into the heart of the city and hiding in a synagogue until the streets became full. Then, they contacted family friends who immediately placed them into hiding. Later that night, their father and mother also successfully escaped Nitra.

So began their new life in an attic in Budapest, which they shared with two other Jewish families. Nana made it her mission to become fluent in Hungarian and was eventually able to obtain fake work papers.

'I dyed my hair blonde and earned money to support the families. I joined the resistance, and we did whatever we could to help other refugees obtain papers or go into hiding. My father and brother left to join the Jewish partisan resistance fighters in the forests near the Slovak–Hungarian border.'

Their life wasn't easy, but it seemed that for now, they had escaped near-certain death and deportation to the concentration camps. Four long years passed. Then, in March 1944, the Nazis invaded Hungary and whispers began circulating about their plan to kill every Jew. Called the 'Final Solution', the nightmare of mass killings and deportations to death camps intensified, and it soon became obvious that the Jews of Budapest were squarely in the Nazis' sights. My grandmother and great-grandmother had jumped from the frying pan into the fire.

With the collaboration of the Hungarian authorities, the Nazis began deporting huge numbers of Jews to the death camps. Within the space of a few months, 434,000 Jews were deported on 147 trains and nearly all of them, men, women and children, were gassed on arrival. The crematoriums were so overwhelmed by the sheer number of bodies that large pits were dug and piles of corpses simply burned. By July 1944, Nana and her mother were among the last remaining Jews in Hungary. They had no idea what to do, and no-one came to help. Nana assumed her father and brother were either still fighting with the resistance or had been killed. They were terrified that the Arrow Cross, the far-right Hungarian fascist party, would find them and shoot them.

'Day after day the Arrow Cross rounded up Jews from the ghettos, lined them up and shot them on the banks of the Danube River. We lost count of how many, but it was in the tens of thousands.'

It reached a point where they felt they had no choice but to try and escape. Nana was friends with a policeman who agreed to escort her and her mother out of the city, but as they made their way through the streets they encountered long lines of emaciated Jews being forcibly marched to their deaths. Decaying bodies littered the roadsides. The sight terrified Nana and her mother so much that they decided to go back to the city and take their chances. Somehow, in the ensuing months, Nana and her mother managed to survive both the Arrow Cross and the Nazis and Allies' intensive bombing of Budapest. When the Soviet army finally liberated Hungary in December 1944, only 70,000 out of the 200,000 Jews who had stayed in the Budapest ghettos were still alive. My Nana and her mum were two of them. Miraculously, a few months after the war ended, Nana was reunited with her father and brother. It was then they learned the fate of their friends and family in Zvolen. Almost everyone they knew had been killed.

Nana closed her eyes, her story complete. I sat in stunned silence for what seemed like minutes before I was able to speak. It was all so incomprehensible to me.

'I can't begin to imagine what you went through. How do you carry on and live a normal life after all that?'

Nana cupped my face in her hands. 'You must understand, Katrinco, the Nazis stole so many years of my life. I vowed not to give them even one more second of my time. If I remained angry and bitter, I'd forever be a victim.'

She was putting words to thoughts and philosophies that had always formed an integral part of my being. I'd inherited not only many of her physical traits but also her innate ability to deal with disaster, to survive it, to move on without lugging emotional baggage into the future.

'Letting go of pain is not forgetting what has been done. I set myself free by putting what happened in another place of my mind. That is why, my darling. I never look backwards. I try to help as many as I can now so they won't have to suffer as I did.'

Whether Nana wanted to accept it or not, she really was a hero in my eyes. Her story allowed me to gain a deeper understanding of her attitude and beliefs around suffering and pain. Because as terrible as the Holocaust was, she viewed her survival as the ultimate triumph of the human spirit over adversity. Even in the depths of despair, when everything of value was taken away from her, she found meaning and purpose in her pain, and this fortified and strengthened her will to live. Perhaps this explained the origin of the power I often felt bubbling up from deep within my soul. Maybe this life force, this determined willpower to survive, was partly a genetic inheritance, passed along by some tough, Jewish matriarchal genes from mother to daughter through the generations.

My grandmother interrupted my thoughts by stating, 'So many of my friends died young, and then when I lost my husband and my daughter—your mother—so close together, there was a part of me that wanted to die too. But I told myself to keep moving forward, to be strong for all of you, to find a purpose within the heartbreak I was experiencing.'

Her stoic words reminded me of a Seneca quote. 'Sometimes, even to live is an act of courage'. Nana's steely will to survive, her choice to leave the past behind and move forward rather than remain a victim, her refusal to give in to the pain and suffering and alternatively transform it—these were actions and behaviours I'd also adopted to survive my disasters. The difference was in the scale and length of suffering my Nana and millions of others like her endured. My disasters paled significantly in comparison.

Her story woke me to the fact I needed to be more grateful and to focus my energy on the things going right rather than the things going wrong. I vowed that if I ever found myself becoming angry, upset or obsessive about any of my relatively insignificant 'First World problems', I'd think about Nana's Holocaust survival and tell myself, 'Stop complaining!'

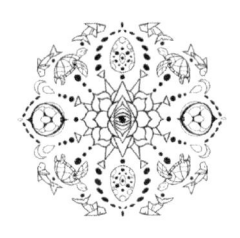

CHAPTER TWENTY-TWO
My First Best Mistake

In life there is 10,000 joys and 10,000 sorrows.
~ Korean proverb

Christmas with my family in Canada was always a festive affair, and this year was no different.

'Happy Hanukkah!' I toasted, raising my glass in acknowledgement of my family's Jewish heritage. Uncle John grinned. In front of him lay a huge Christmas feast, including a large ham.

'Oh great. If you're converting, that means more pork for me,' he said, rubbing his hands gleefully.

If my father could be described as a sarcastic, grimly hilarious man, my uncle John was his maniacal twin. Nana's story had given my siblings and I fresh insight into our heritage and a better understanding of how our grandmother had gained her indomitable strength of spirit. I liked to think some of this strength had been passed on to us, as we were adept at soldiering on in the face of life's tougher challenges.

'Hey, by the way, Nana says to wish all of you a Merry Christmas,' I announced. 'She's at Uncle Paul's for the holidays this year. Could you please pass me the ham? It looks delicious.'

There was only one thing missing from the Christmas celebrations, as far as I was concerned, and it wasn't Twizzlers. It was Trev. He was firmly wedged in my mind and my heart. I was aching to be back with him, even if it meant returning to Jrudgerie. Surely now, after getting the wanderlust out of my system and having so many European adventures, I could live in a small town and be happy. Hell, after what my grandmother and her family had to deal with, Jrudgerie should be a cinch!

Trev and I had been in constant contact since I'd left Australia six months earlier. We'd concluded that despite time and distance we still deeply loved each other. It seemed our love was a boomerang after all. The good news was, Trev had been working steadily on the reno of his grandfather's cottage and hoped to finish it soon. He planned to rent it, then move to the coast. I could have both my man and my dream life on the beach if I went back.

So I bought yet another ticket to Australia, much to the amusement of my father, and again travelled several days to reach the edge of the outback and settle into the back of beyond. I was able to work with Trevor doing some painting. My skills had now improved enough that I was trusted to do more than just wall washing and sanding. To supplement the painting income, I taught aerobics, aqua fit and swimming lessons at the local community centre in the evenings and on weekends. I also turned my hand to gardening and sowing beds full of seasonal vegetables. I didn't bother planting fruit trees, though. I figured I'd be long gone before they produced their first crop.

Four months after arriving in Jrudgerie I began feeling unwell. This time it wasn't my arm or shoulder. Rather, I felt nauseated on an almost daily basis, especially in the mornings. I was no stranger to hangovers, but this was different, and I doubted a Berocca would cure what I had. It was ANZAC day, a national holiday in Australia held in remembrance of those who died in war. Trev was playing in the annual Jrudgerie golf tournament. As per usual, nearly the entire town showed up to take part in the event. All the shops were shut, and the only pharmacy open was nearly an hour's drive in a tourist town on the mighty Murray River. I made up an excuse to Trev about why I suddenly didn't want to play golf, and during the drive I reflected on how fortunate it was I wouldn't be buying the pregnancy test locally. If I had, the whole town would gossip about us and people would constantly look at my belly for telltale signs.

I arrived at the pharmacy, purchased my pregnancy test and walked out to my car. Yes, I was safe, my secret intact. Then a car swung into the space next to me. I heard my name being yelled out. I looked up and realised it was Shae, Trev's sister. You've got to be kidding! Of all the people in the world to bump into on a secret pregnancy run, why her? Shae had an uncanny ability to read me like a book and an unnerving ability to predict the future. She slid out of the car, smiling brightly and asked what

I was doing so far from home. My brain froze. I told her I was buying lollies and held up the paper bag as evidence. She looked at me suspiciously. In the background, I heard her kids yell, 'Yay, lollies!'

'Hmmm, well I just bought some fresh doughnuts. Want to come to the farm for some tea?'

I didn't want tea; I wanted to pee on a stick. But I couldn't say no—she was already looking at me quizzically.

I jumped in my car and managed to arrive at the farm first. Mercifully, nobody in that part of the world locked their doors. I raced into the house ahead of Shae and went straight to the loo, tore open the box with the magic stick and peed on it. When I saw the second red line appear I realised my future was sealed. I was pregnant!

I swung open the door. Shae was standing on the other side, her daughter Bella nestled on her hip. White with shock, I thrust the stick into her hand and begged her to tell me I was mistaken. She glanced at it, laughed with happiness and pulled me into a tight, one-armed hug. Bella tapped me on the shoulder, asking if she could have a lolly. I didn't know whether to laugh, cry or vomit.

I returned to Jrudgerie in the afternoon, a million thoughts swirling round in my head. Trev and I had been dating on and off for a few years and hadn't seriously discussed parenthood or marriage. I was mulling over how to break the news to him when he bounded through the front door, picked me up and spun me around.

'We won the golf!'

He was clearly well on his way into his celebrations. 'I've just run home to grab some cash for a few more beers.'

I knew it wasn't the best time, but I've never been one to hide the truth for long. I decided to break the news to him subtly. I closed my eyes, took a deep breath and blurted, 'You're going to be a dad!'

When I opened my eyes, the expression on his face was priceless. I needn't have worried—he was elated. In fact, he was so excited, he dropped to his knees, held my hips and started talking to my belly. As he chatted with the developing embryo I heard a car pull up.

'It's your mother.'

Before I could stop him he was off like a shot, opening her car door and animatedly telling her she was going to be a grandma. He then ran the 500 metres to the golf club and announced it to the entire community.

'Drinks on me! I'm going to be a dad!'

But the next morning, when the alcohol gave way to the cold light of day, he woke up and decided he wasn't ready to be a father. I was seriously pissed off—not because of his uncertainty but because he'd changed his mind after telling the world.

For the next few weeks I agonised about what to do. I was 26, old enough to have known better than to land myself in this situation but overcome with a protective maternal instinct. I was in love with the idea of a baby growing inside me.

Trevor's family knew we were expecting, but they also knew he wasn't sold on the idea. My closest friends in town were his mother and sisters. It was an awful time for me as Trevor wavered daily about how he felt, leaving me grappling with the decision of whether to stay or go back to Canada and do parenthood alone. It was awkward to say the least. Finally, he came around and embraced the idea of impending fatherhood.

In six weeks we were married. It was an intimate affair, just his family, a few friends, my dad and stepmother. My siblings wanted to be there, but I suggested they come another time. It was a lot of money to travel to a shotgun wedding in the middle of a Melbourne winter. Despite their absence, our wedding was perfect. Six months later and two days before Christmas, I went into labour in a small country hospital a hundred kilometres from Jrudgerie. The one person who I had fought with the most growing up, my perfect sister Wendy, was by my side. She'd flown all the way from Canada to be with us. It meant the world to me. Trev was there too for the entire 16 hours of labour, although he thought nothing about complaining he had wet shoes after helping me in the shower. I had chosen a natural birth with no pain relief other than gas—no needles for me, especially an epidural in my back! I gave birth to a baby boy. We named him Jack.

Our little Jack-a-roo was perfect in every way. He slept when he was supposed to and cried only when hungry. I'd never known this kind of love before. This tiny baby held my whole heart. I swore I'd never leave him. Everything was going right in my world. I had a perfect little boy, a loving extended Aussie family, a sister by my side, and a husband who not only loved me but also adored our new baby. And thanks to playing host to a human parasite, I lost my weight as quickly as Jack gained his. My belly was the flattest it had ever been, and for once, I even had a chest to be proud of. Three weeks after giving birth I was teaching fitness classes, looking curvaceous and feeling great.

But then something weird happened: I started getting tired—not just a little tired, a lot tired. Thinking was an effort. I could barely move from the couch. It was even hard for me to do up the snaps on the baby clothes. For someone like me, used to being the Energiser Bunny, an unstoppable force with boundless energy, this was highly unusual. Unfortunately, my sister had just left. She'd been not only my moral support and confidant during and after the birth but also a welcome helping hand with the baby.

A few days later I started tripping over. When I tried to put on my left shoe, I found I couldn't. My leg wouldn't lift. That bloody psychic and my left leg! She'd really nailed it. I intuited almost immediately that the symptoms which had once debilitated my right arm had come back—only this time they had migrated to my leg. It was time to see Dr Alphabet again. I prayed he could give me a course of steroids and once again magically cure me.

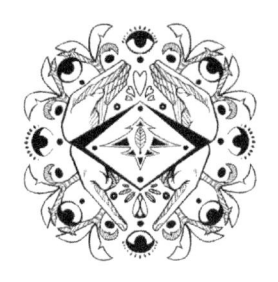

CHAPTER TWENTY-THREE
A Slippery Slope into a Black Hole

Black holes ain't as black as they are painted to be. They are not the eternal prisons they were once thought. Things can get out of a black hole, both on the outside, and possibly, to another universe. So, if you feel you are in a black hole, don't give up. There's a way out.
~ Stephen Hawking

The last time I saw Dr Alphabet was two years prior, when my right arm stopped working. At the time he explained the problem was a result of inflammation. The insulation around my nerves was being attacked, most likely due to an auto-immune reaction. When the steroid treatment worked like a charm and I felt almost as good as new, I'd been confident it would never happen to me again. Except, of course, now it had.

I rang Dr Alphabet. After exchanging pleasantries and informing him I'd just had a baby, I described my symptoms. He hesitated before answering.

'Kat...look, I'm sorry to have to tell you this, but when you have more than one attack of this kind, our diagnosis changes. Based on previous tests and the symptoms you're describing, I'm fairly certain you have a serious auto-immune disease called multiple sclerosis, otherwise known as MS.'

MS? Wait, wasn't that the same disease the woman in the wheelchair had at the bachelor auction all those years ago? But... but that was an incurable illness, a death sentence, a one-way ticket to a nursing home.

I refocused on my neuro, who was still talking: 'We can start treatment straight away. I'll meet you at the emergency department of the Alfred Hospital this evening.'

My mother-in-law was holding my hand during the call. When I hung up she let go and hugged me tightly as I broke down and sobbed. The tears were not just for me but for my baby. I didn't want my only son to grow up having to look after me. A horrible vision of myself paralysed, slumped in a wheelchair being fed by my child formed in my mind. I forced it away.

I called Trevor at work. He came home straight away so we could organise the four-hour trip to Melbourne with our newborn in tow. While waiting for him to arrive, I called the MS Society to gain some clarity about what I was dealing with. The number rang once, then went straight to a pre-recorded message.

'MS is a chronic, progressive disease that strikes young people down in the prime of their life.'

I slammed the phone down, glaring at it. That was not going to be me. I refused to be struck down by anything.

The amazing Dr Alphabet was waiting for me at the Alfred Hospital in Melbourne when we arrived. As usual, he was incredibly kind, caring and compassionate. He'd organised for me to go into a room without having to wait in the emergency area. He sat with me for over an hour. I think maybe he was concerned I was in shock or denial because I was so calm about everything. But the truth was, I'd had six hours to process the diagnosis, accept it and move on. I reassured him I was fine.

He explained it was his duty to inform me about my illness. He described exactly how MS was damaging the myelin sheath around my nerves. How my body's own immune cells, which were normally supposed to protect me from disease by attacking anything foreign in my blood, had crossed the blood–brain barrier and were now attacking the nerve cells in my central nervous system instead. I envisioned a plague of miniature rats chewing away on electrical cords, causing parts of the house to short circuit and go black. I didn't want to think about it.

I looked down at Jack, sleeping soundly in my arms. And then I asked Dr Alphabet the only thing I wanted to know.

'What are the chances of my child contracting MS?'

'Ah…right…of course. Well, you have no family history of multiple sclerosis, so chances are slim your baby will inherit this.'

I breathed a sigh of relief.

'I mean, there's a small amount of genetic predisposition or heritability, but there are other contributing factors, like smoking, childhood obesity, contracting glandular fever or herpes, even a lack of vitamin D.'

'Well at least I have control over the last one,' I said in mock relief. 'I have no problems at all ensuring my baby and I live a life of perpetual summer.'

'Look, Kat, the point is, MS is a progressive disease and there's no cure. I'm sorry to tell you, but patients with your type of relapsing-remitting MS always deteriorate over time. Attacks will eventually become more frequent and more debilitating and often lead to secondary progressive MS.'

I wanted to plug my ears and scream, 'Stop! Don't tell me any more,' but I forced myself to stay calm and in control. It took a supreme amount of willpower to do this.

'The good news is, there are a few different drugs available. They're all delivered by self-injection. Sometimes they can reduce the relapse rate by around 30 per cent.'

How could he call this good news? It meant 70 percent of attacks would still occur even after I'd tortured myself with injections.

'We'll start you on a four-day course of steroids to dampen your immune response, reduce inflammation and hopefully fix your leg. You'll receive the first one here in the hospital. After that, a nurse will come to where you're staying in Melbourne to administer the next three. Then you'll need to go directly on to the disease-modifying injections.'

He added somewhat optimistically, 'With the right treatment regime we should be able to keep you walking unassisted until at least the age of 40.'

Somehow he made it sound like this was a win. But there was more bad news to come. He went on to advise me not to have any more children, noting that while pregnancy seemed to provide some protection against relapses, the flip side was that after giving birth the likelihood of having a severe attack increased substantially.

'So you should be happy with your one healthy little boy.'

I was quiet, not quite sure how to take this.

'Oh, and I'm very sorry to tell you, but once we begin the steroid infusion and you start on the disease-modifying therapy, you won't be able to breastfeed.'

He must have noticed the look of despair on my face because he asked, 'Are you okay?'

In my head I screamed, 'No!' but somehow kept it together and nodded. I held back the tears that threatened to fall as I cradled Jack in my right arm while I watched them insert the cannula into my left arm. The nurse cleared the lines and hooked up the methylprednisolone. My heart ached as I looked at my little angel. He smiled and finished feeding from me for the last time. As Jack drifted off into a peaceful slumber, Trev left to buy baby formula and bottles. I tried to sleep.

Jack woke up an hour later. Contented at first, he eventually transitioned to crying and then to full-blown wailing like only a hungry newborn can. Unfortunately, I couldn't feed him due to the steroids coursing through my veins. I tried my best to settle him with one arm attached to an IV pole. We were in a cubicle partially curtained off from the rest of the ER, and people began staring at me, some with sympathy, others with thinly disguised irritation. Many were no doubt wondering, 'Why don't you feed that baby?' But there was nothing I could do. I knew the last thing anyone needed in the emergency room was a screaming child. Where the hell was Trevor? I was furious! It seemed like an eternity before a kind nurse finally managed to obtain a bottle of formula from the maternity ward and present it to Jack. He took to it like a cowboy to beer, then burped and fell back to sleep.

Trevor eventually returned, baby bottles in hand and beer on his breath. He apologised for taking so long, admitting he'd stopped at a pub for a quick pint and a bite to eat. I was ropeable. All I could think of was how selfish and inconsiderate he'd been. At the time I never considered what he must have been going through. My perception was that I was the one suffering, I was the one with the baby and the disease. Trev was healthy and free.

Four days later, after completing the steroid treatment, I made a conscious decision to defy the doctor's orders and delay the injections of beta interferon, the disease-modifying drug. I wanted to continue to breastfeed my baby. I couldn't bring myself to break the mother-child bond. More importantly, I was a believer in all things natural, and my priority was to give my baby the best possible start in life.

I returned to Jrudgerie unsure of what lay ahead. By now my left leg had improved dramatically, and I could almost walk without limping. The limb seemed to be following the same recovery trajectory as my right arm had years earlier. Dr Alphabet did say that the body could repair itself to some extent during the earlier stages of MS. The brain could reroute itself around damaged nerves in a process known as 'plasticity', and the myelin sheath could regrow around the damaged nerves, although it tended to grow back thinner. The only drawback? Messages from the brain to the limbs would invariably slow down.

I was actually feeling pretty good by the time I strolled into the local doctor's office for my six-week postpartum check-up. I knew all the girls in the reception, many of whom were participants in my aerobics classes. We greeted each other warmly. I walked into my GP's office with Jack cradled in my arms and handed over the letter from my neurologist outlining my diagnosis and treatment. She read it and looked up at me in shock.

'Oh Kat, I'm so sorry. How are you feeling?'

'I'm okay, I'm feeling good,' I said smiling, absentmindedly rocking Jack gently in my arms.

She glanced at the baby and looked back at me. I saw her eyes well up.

'I, um, I just need to go out and put this in your file at reception,' she said, her voice breaking a little. She was back a few minutes later, composed and professional, and completed my check-up.

I found out many years later that when she'd stepped out for those few minutes and reached the reception desk she couldn't contain her tears. One of the nurses glanced at the neuro's report the doctor had given her to file and showed it to the rest of the staff. They were all extremely upset. And there I was sitting in the office happily singing to my baby boy, oblivious to the tears being shed for me. This was something I would have to deal with more and more as people found out about my illness. Their reactions often far exceeded mine. Strange as it may seem, I didn't think having MS was worth the pity and the fuss, and I refused to wear the diagnosis. My mantra was, 'I'm perfectly fine, there's nothing wrong with me! I will not worry or think about symptoms that have not happened yet.'

Maybe this was just part of my personality—I'm a very practical person from a very practical family—or maybe most people with a similar life-changing diagnosis go through this rationalisation process. Either way, I didn't like to dwell on my problems and hated being pitied almost as much as I disliked seeing people wallow in self-pity. Basically, it came down to a perception issue. If I gave my diagnosis an identity, a story, then very quickly it would engulf me and morph into a destiny I did not want to manifest. I figured I could help shape my reality by changing my perception of it, and this in turn would change my experience of MS and eventually change me.

Eight months later I stopped breastfeeding Jack. I was now ready to begin the beta interferon drug therapy, delivered via self-injection every other day. I was reminded interferon was a powerful drug that could cause various side effects, including depression, flu-like symptoms and itchy, red skin around the injection site. I didn't care about the side effects, but the prospect of daily injections freaked me out. I refused to inject myself. As a result, Trev derived great pleasure playing doctor by jabbing needles into my butt. Did the drug help? I wasn't entirely convinced but admittedly wasn't able to give it much of a chance. After only two months I was forced to go off it. I'd accidentally fallen pregnant again. Oops!

My second son, Luke, was born in June the following year. As the neurologist warned, I quickly went downhill. I had two MS attacks within the first six months of Luke's birth, resulting in both my left arm and right leg losing dexterity, strength and coordination. MS had now left no limbs untouched. I was admitted for progressive rounds of steroid infusions. I recovered, but the attacks were beginning to have lasting effects. Nevertheless, I was once again committed to breastfeeding my baby and held off resuming the beta interferon drug therapy.

Luke was 18 months old when we sang 'Happy Birthday' to Jack on his third birthday. He blew out the three candles on his Ninja Turtles cake. As for me, I was heavily pregnant once again. Four days later, our third and final Oops was born, this time a beautiful baby girl, Stella. She was the perfect gift of happiness and joy. Yes, I know what you're thinking. How could anyone be so stupid as to have three unplanned pregnancies in three years, especially following a diagnosis of MS? I couldn't agree more, but suffice it to say, there were extenuating circumstances. And not once did I regret having any of my children. Every one of my kids turned out to be flaxen-haired and blue-eyed. Damn that clairvoyant—first the left leg, now the kids—she'd earned every penny of her 20 bucks.

A few days after giving birth to Stella, I checked us out of the hospital and drove the 150 km home. On the way I grocery shopped, got a speeding ticket and, after arriving, cooked dinner for our now family of five. I refused to let my circumstances slow me down. As we sat down to eat there was a knock on the door. It was Trevor's cousin, Brad, who dropped in from time to time for an all-night drinking session. He never called ahead even though he lived four hours away. Trev was very excited to see him. Brad insisted on taking him out for a few beers to 'wet the baby's head'. Trevor gave us all a kiss goodbye before going off to celebrate, leaving me home alone at the end of a very long day with a three-year-old, an 18-month-old and a three-day-old crying baby. I wanted to flush Trev's head down the toilet.

Okay, I wasn't entirely blameless in this scenario. Trev wasn't running off with Brad because he couldn't cope with the idea of having another baby. Rather, it was because Trev had an unflappable belief in my ability to handle anything. I was strong-willed and too proud to ever admit I was suffering. Whenever someone asked how I was going or if I needed help, I'd say, 'I'm good, I've got this.' And most of the time; it was true. But the reality was, I was now a mother to three very young children and had a progressive, debilitating disease with no known cure. My carefree existence of just 36 months prior had disappeared. I was married to a painter who lived in the middle of nowhere and, ironically, it seemed I had painted myself into a corner. How in hell was I ever going to get myself out?

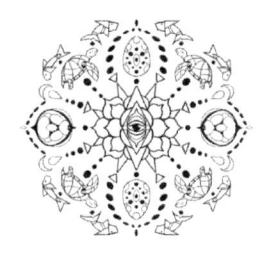

CHAPTER TWENTY-FOUR
The Blissful Pursuit of Ignorance

If ignorance is bliss, why aren't more people happy?
~ Thomas Jefferson

In the weeks following Stella's birth, Dr Alphabet's warning kept echoing in my head. There was now a very good possibility I would relapse in the next few months. It was time to stop being a martyr and a hero and ask for help. But did I do that? No. I went back to work teaching fitness classes when Stella was just three weeks old, partly because I didn't want to lose my sense of self and partly because I wanted to prove to myself I could still do anything I set my mind to. Each morning, after a night of minimal sleep, I'd breastfeed my newborn and then dress two wild toddlers and myself simultaneously so I could be out of the house by 8 a.m. to teach classes. Pure madness.

It wasn't surprising when I suffered another attack three months later. This one was far more severe than the previous ones. It took away the function of my left leg again, which was mentally devastating for me as it had only just partially recovered thanks to earlier steroid treatments. The attack also distorted the vision in my left eye. I think maybe it was a sign from God, telling me to stop being so blind.

I now walked like a young version of Stephen Hawking. My left leg dragged and my left foot flopped awkwardly, crippled by a condition known as drop foot. Together, they caused me to sway, trip constantly and lean perpetually to the right like the tower of Pisa. This no doubt contributed to my scoliosis, a curvature of the spine in my lower back, which I developed later in life. Despite my ever-growing list of disabilities, I refused to give up. I was desperately trying to hold everything together. But I was losing the battle.

Some say there's no disgrace in failing, in being vulnerable, imperfect. That showing humility and reaching out for help is not a sign of weakness but of true courage and strength. That sharing the burden of suffering gives others the opportunity to foster deeper connections, meaning and purpose, provided it's done from a position of need rather than from a misguided bid for attention or pity. Humility and vulnerability can be a wonderful gift when shared with the right intentions, not just for others around you but also for yourself.

Pride and ego prevented me from asking for help or even admitting I wasn't coping. And although I knew from my army days this was a potential weakness, I ignored those lessons to my detriment. Instead, I attempted a delicate balancing act: on the one hand, trying to keep my mind and body strong, and on the other, hoping I would have enough fortitude and energy to stay in control of the situation. But having three children in three years meant I'd piled immense pressure on myself and my body. Like Papa Joe used to say, 'You make your choices, then your choices make you.'

Eight months after Stella was born I stopped breastfeeding and begrudgingly went back on the 'disease-modifying' injections. I'd had multiple attacks in the interim, and although I knew the drugs were never going to be a cure, I still hoped they would delay the progression long enough to buy me enough time to find one.

My new mission was to prevent more attacks from occurring and strengthen my body and mind to support the broken bits of me. I began a strict therapeutic diet, ate loads of vegetables, avoided dairy, meat and all saturated fats, exercised daily and made sure I overdosed on plenty of natural and liquid vitamin D. I consumed a steady diet of self-help books, absorbing all relevant information I could find, collating anything that resonated with my beliefs and adapting it to my lifestyle. I disassociated myself from my diagnosis and avoided support groups like I avoided sitting on public toilet seats or going to the mall on Boxing Day. I wasn't interested in seeing what could happen to me or listening to others sharing their endless problems of woe. When I had MRIs, I refused to hear the results. I didn't want proof of the damage MS was inflicting on my central nervous system.

This wasn't an act of stupidity. I was mindfully maintaining a blissful pursuit of ignorance. My results wouldn't change my reality, and I knew my condition was worsening, but I didn't need the evidence shoved in my face, causing me more stress and creating a nasty feedback loop. The only time I went to a doctor was when I was under attack and had lost the use of a body part. I spent a fair amount of time in waiting rooms and hospitals.

I embraced everything natural but knew I couldn't completely shun Western medicine. When you suddenly lose the ability to walk, nothing works as fast or is more welcome than a massive hit of steroids. Drugs can be your best friend, but inevitably, that which brings you instant happiness can also bring you long-term pain. I call it the karmic law of pharmaceuticals. And for me, the drugs that helped me through the hardest times came at a high price. Many years of steroid use would eventually take their toll on my body—in particular, the deterioration of the vertebrae in my spine.

In the meantime life continued on regardless of my health issues. One of the benefits of having a well-to-do Jewish grandmother who loved being surrounded by her family was she subsidised our annual trips to Canada from Australia. We had no mortgage hanging over our heads, thanks to our house being worth less than a moderately priced second-hand German car, so taking extended holidays wasn't an issue for us as a family.

The Canada trips proved to be a bonus for the kids as well as for me. They grew up knowing both sides of the family and were able to experience the magic of a white, snowy Christmas in Toronto. And I was given the break I desperately needed from life in Jrudgerie. We based ourselves at my Dad's house. Most of my siblings were still living at home and those who weren't came back for holidays. When you added in the five of us, it meant there were often 11 people living under one roof. My family would brace themselves for our arrival. Dad rechristened my boys Search and Destroy because they were like unguided missiles, wrecking everything in their path. Stella, on the other hand, was the most delightfully perfect human. She obviously took after my sister Wendy.

I loved these times in Canada with my family. Unlike when I was a child, I now craved the company of my brother and sisters. My heart overflowed with joy whenever we were together. I felt unbelievably blessed to be part of such a large, loving family. But as much as Trevor enjoyed spending time with all of us in Canada, he always wanted to return to his own family and home in Jrudgerie. Understandable, of course. And although I absolutely adored Trev's family, whenever it came time for us to leave Canada, a deep sadness would overwhelm me. Toronto was my home. It was where my heart and my family were. But we had our businesses and a life back in Australia, and despite the MS, I continued to push myself hard. In the end, something had to give. And that something was me.

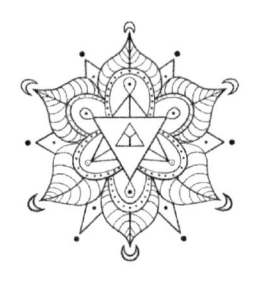

CHAPTER TWENTY-FIVE
The Miracle of Spandex

Each day, each moment, you have a choice to either do things that will make your body and mind stronger or weaker. There are only two choices, no in-between. Ask yourself from moment to moment, what would my future self want me to do right now?
Then live your life by this principle.
~ Connor MacLaren

I heard a loud snap and knew I'd finally pushed myself too far as I tripped over the step and cracked my head into the brick wall behind me. I was halfway through teaching a 6 a.m. step class at the Jrudgerie Sports Centre. My dodgy left leg hadn't lifted high enough, causing me to lose my balance and wrench my ankle.

At this point I'd had MS for just over five years, and nearly every exercise I once found easy was now challenging. I coped by modifying my routines and reminding myself over and over to just find another way, keep going no matter what. I was constantly playing a game of cat and mouse with the thoughts in my head. Sometimes I'd think, *This is embarrassing, I can't run or lift my leg, and here I am trying to teach exercise classes.* Then my gritty side would kick in and I'd tell myself, 'Stop it, stay strong. Find a way!'

I finished the class by calling out the steps, then hobbled to the doctor in Jrudgerie to deal with my rapidly swelling ankle. I suspected it was fractured, as my leg was beginning to go purple from the knee down. The timing was terrible. It was five days before Christmas, I had yet to do any gift shopping and I was facing the prospect of spending the summer in a cast and on crutches. It was time to pack the step away and find another way to work and stay fit.

As it turned out, I had an avulsion fracture. My tendon had ripped a piece of bone from my ankle. The good news was, I didn't need surgery, just a few weeks in a moon boot. I did my best to rest my leg, but the word relax wasn't in my vocabulary. With a business to run and children to mind, I concluded the only way I'd get better was to take a trip home to Canada with Stella, the only kid I didn't have to chase after. Maybe I could also improve my balance by trying yoga at the local gym.

The idea of yoga intrigued me, however my one and only experience of it had been entirely unsatisfying. A few years earlier, while I was in Canada on one of our extended family trips, I was working out at the gym with my friend when she suggested trying a yoga class. I figured with all the people walking around in Lululemon leggings, it couldn't be that bad. It turned out I was wrong. I hated it! The teacher was a middle-aged, waif-like blonde with a breathy, spaced-out voice who spoke using obscure yoga terms. In between painful stretches we did repetitive sun salutations, where we rose and fell to the floor like demented marionettes. She murmured about blocked chakras and Ananda bliss and encouraged us to chant. I was out of there before they finished the first 'om'.

This time I was on a mission to give yoga another chance. The fact the new yoga teacher at my gym was a chiselled, good-looking South African guy in tight spandex may have slightly influenced my decision. My first class with Joshua was nothing like my previous yoga experience. For a start, the sessions were three hours long, fast-paced and challenging. He had us doing postures and movements I'd never encountered before. This wasn't relaxation with a few stretches; it was a full-blown mind and body awakening! I called it yoga on steroids. I did my best to complete all the movements despite the limits imposed upon my body by the MS and my slowly healing left ankle. By the time meditation came around I was supremely grateful to lie down and surrender into *savasana*, the aptly named 'corpse pose', which Joshua explained was not only for relaxation but also meant we symbolically 'died' to our unhelpful ways of thinking.

After only a few sessions with my new yoga teacher I started to feel my body become stronger, more balanced, flexible and coordinated. But it was the changes to my mind that really blew me away. I felt like each yoga session was a cleaning of my mental house, retraining my brain to talk to my body in new ways. I felt refreshed, reborn and empowered. Yoga gave me the same sense of happiness as a couple of glasses of bubbly, except when I practised yoga I could walk straighter and had no hangover or regrets the next day! I soon became as addicted to yoga with Joshua as I was to champagne. And my ankle healed in record time. Eventually, however, I had to return to Australia and leave Joshua's well-spandexed behind…behind.

Back in Jrudgerie, I incorporated some of Joshua's yoga routines into my fitness classes. It proved to be popular and beneficial not just for my clients but for me as well. I suffered fewer injuries and my balance and strength improved. And six months after that I was once again back in Toronto, busting to recommence yoga sessions with my old teacher. But I was told by the gym staff that Joshua had moved on and been replaced by an instructor named Connor. I was crushed. Who the hell was this Connor guy? How dare he replace my Joshua! I prayed he was as skilled a teacher as my chiselled South African and, more importantly, looked as good in spandex.

I turned up to the yoga session the following day and noticed a big line-up of people waiting to enter, mats in hand. I joined the queue, curious about the excitement. When I entered the room I was surprised and mystified by the appearance of the new teacher. Not only was Connor a stocky, kind of studious-looking guy with auburn hair and thick Coke-bottle glasses, but he was dressed in cargo pants and a button-up shirt! Where were the tight spandex pants and exposed rippling torso? He was definitely no Joshua! More importantly, how the hell was he going to teach us wearing those clothes? I found a space next to the wall and apprehensively rolled out my mat.

There must have been at least 50 of us crammed into a room meant to fit 30, everyone staking out their own little piece of yoga real estate. And yet the moment Connor commenced his yoga session there was absolute silence. That was when I began to suspect this guy was a true yoga master, although I doubt he'd ever refer to himself as one. He seemed to command complete respect from his students without ego. He radiated an aura of calm assurance. He led the class by speaking in plain English, only rarely throwing in the odd yoga term as he casually walked around observing each student with the eye of a master. He spoke infrequently, and when he did, we listened. It was a power yoga class, but ten minutes in I thought they should have renamed it the torture yoga class. It was insanely challenging.

What I found even harder to comprehend was that Connor rarely did the postures himself. Rather, he walked around and guided us with precise verbal instructions. Very occasionally he showed us how to do a pose but would immediately go back to moving around the room. He had us holding postures and stretches for so long that our muscles started to shake, our arms and legs gave way and many of us collapsed onto the ground in total agony. When we reached these points where we thought we couldn't possibly go on, Connor would casually stroll past and say something utterly pragmatic but insightful.

'Yoga is about existing in the moment. Find and centre yourself in your breath as you calmly face your challenge head-on and learn how to control life's stressful situations through practice.'

Or sometimes he would intone in a soft, steady voice, 'The intensity of this physical and emotional pain will eventually pass, but it's how you respond and react to that pain in the moment that really counts. In this class you can choose to stop whenever you want, but remember, unless you challenge yourself, you will never create change. Your comfort zone is a nice place to live, but there's no growth there.'

It soon became apparent that these 'Connorisms', as I called them, applied equally well to the painful and challenging situations in my everyday life as well as on the yoga mat. One of my biggest tests was balancing on one leg. My balance was pretty horrific even with two feet planted firmly on the ground, but trying to do a tree pose on a semi-paralysed left leg had me wobbling like a drunken schoolgirl. I was always careful to position myself next to a wall in any class so I could hang on to it for dear life. I did the best I could, even when it seemed pointless. But after literally thousands of failed attempts, my brain and body started finding a way. I began experiencing small but consistent improvements. Connor was life-changing for me, not only as an insightful yoga teacher but also because his philosophy, life history and attitude resonated with me. I felt like we were kindred spirits. He taught me not to be ignorant of any tiny improvement. He used to say, 'With wisdom comes knowledge. When we ignore knowledge we are ignorant, we are ignoring the facts.'

I could not ignore the fact that my body and mind were becoming wiser, stronger, more connected. My thoughts were becoming more peaceful every time I finished a yoga session. What I found incomprehensible was why this kind of intensive body and brain re-training wasn't prescribed to all MS patients. I'd never been offered any physio training during my MS journey, even while suffering from the worst of my attacks. The general consensus seemed to be that it would make little difference to my recovery. My experience with yoga proved this was fundamentally wrong, at least for me. Plus, it had the added benefit of making me mentally strong and reducing stress, and this in turn seemed to stop all my symptoms from escalating. So I studied to be a yoga teacher and incorporated Connor's movements and philosophies into my own classes. I committed myself to spreading the word and helping people heal.

During times of sporadic hospitalisation after severe MS attacks, I'd use my newfound yoga skills and Connor's philosophy about overcoming challenges to help me through the hard times. Quite often the ward nurses would find me doing stretches on my yoga mat or holding a warrior pose or doing sun salutations while hooked up to an IV. Some would smile encouragingly, but occasionally a nurse would admonish me.

'You're sick, you should be resting.'

To which I'd counter, 'I'm not sick. I'm getting treatment, but I am not sick!'

Nothing raises my hackles more than someone placing a label on me and then telling me I should relax and take it easy. I wanted to scream, 'That's the last thing I should be doing! Can't you see I'm doing what I need to do to stay healthy?!'

I repeated Connor's favourite sayings in my head whenever times got tough:

'You have a choice when dealing with painful challenges, give up or push past it.'

'The longer you focus on the pain, the worse it becomes.'

'Breathe through it, tell yourself a new story.'

'This is where the growth happens.'

'Like all things in life, this too will pass.'

These were mantras for my mind and my body. When the doctors at the hospital checked my medical chart, they'd remark how well I was responding to various treatments.

'This drug would flatten most other patients,' they'd say.

I'd enthusiastically tell them about yoga and the power of the mind. They'd nod, make some encouraging comments, then move on, dismissing what I had to say because it didn't fit into their neat scientific box. I don't think they grasped the fact that yoga wasn't just about touching your toes; it was about everything you discovered on the way down. It meant learning how to bend and not break through the application of flexibility, balance, openness, and patience on both a physical and mental level. I often wondered, if the health system cared as much about the mind and body remaining healthy, strong and in tune while going through treatments for disease or illness as it did about prescribing pharmaceutical drugs, would the outcomes for recovery be radically different?

Despite knowing all this and recognising that yoga was one of the most powerful tools in my arsenal for keeping my mind and body strong. I stopped practising it when I began spiralling into depression six months later. Funny how we often sabotage ourselves even though we know better.

CHAPTER TWENTY-SIX
A Cry For Help

You cannot force out the darkness or try to sweep it away because it will only be replaced by more darkness. You can only bring in the light.
~ Elizabeth Gilbert

It was now 2006, and life in my little outback Aussie town was no longer dull but hectic as all hell. In addition to being a mother to three little people, I was now president of the preschool and running the Council Sports Centre with the help of a partner. I conducted community weight-loss and wellness classes, wrote nutrition and fitness articles for the local paper and taught healing and nutrition with whole food cooking classes. I refused to let MS slow me down. I was constantly generating new ideas, which kept me busy and focused and stopped me from dwelling on my worsening health situation. It also meant I was burning the candle at both ends. Some might say I was my own worst enemy, pushing my body well past its limits, but I never saw it that way.

Living with MS meant dealing with a continuous cycle of relapses and remissions. I never knew what would happen next. There were many times I'd wake up and parts of my body no longer worked. Often I was physically unable to teach an aerobics class, so I'd disguise my inability to function by setting up a circuit and instructing from the sidelines. I became a master at hiding the extent of my progressing disabilities. For example, if my legs weren't working properly, I'd put my toddler in a stroller that doubled as a walking frame before going outside.

The disease attacked different areas of my body at different times and in different ways. Even the simplest actions became challenging, like using a knife and fork when my hands were weakened. Outside my home, I tried to act as though everything was great. I had too much pride to admit to anyone how bad I was getting. But inside, things were quickly falling apart. I was not coping and constantly descended into a mental hell of rage and frustration over everything I was losing. My suffering was compounded by my inability to see all that was good in my life.

Each day I bided my time, waiting for it to end so I could finally tuck the kids into bed and cuddle up next to them, reading their favourite books. But the optic neuritis caused by my MS obscured the vision in my left eye and turned even this fleetingly happy time into a cruel reminder that my life was going downhill. I was trying hard to be a somebody—a mother, a wife, a businesswoman—when all I wanted to do was drift off and be a nobody.

I started taking my frustrations out on Trev. I felt like he was the lucky one, going off to work every day, then coming home to drink a few beers, relax on the couch, play a bit with the kids, and disappear into his shed. Saying I was bitter would be an understatement. I focused on all the bad things and had a difficult time seeing the good. In truth, he was a hard worker, kind-hearted and a great father to our kids. He was doing the best he could and coping in his own way.

There was one incident I'll never forget. It highlighted my worsening relationship with my husband, my deteriorating attitude towards life and my stubborn refusal to face reality. It was the summer holidays, and we'd rented a house for a week on the coast. Every morning we were greeted by schools of dolphins surfing the waves. I decided to take a walk down the beach with the kids one beautiful sunny morning. They were three, four and five years old at the time.

I knew if my body became overheated it would affect the ability of my damaged demyelinated nerves to conduct electrical impulses, resulting in a temporary worsening of every past symptom. But it was a cool morning, and I dismissed the danger. I lost myself in the joy of the moment, playing with the kids and walking way too far. When the heat intensified, my legs stopped working properly. I fell to the sand, unable to move, a tiny, white, beached whale stranded by the outgoing tide.

It broke my heart when little Stella knelt in the sand next to me and reassured me, 'Don't worry Mummy, it'll be okay. I can carry you.'

I smiled at her but in my head was screaming, 'No, *I'm* the one who's meant to carry *you*!'

I dragged my body to the water's edge and tried to cool myself off in order to regain a semblance of movement. It helped a little. My three kids then half-carried, half-dragged me all the way back. Concerned passers-by asked us if we needed help. I waved them away, smiling and saying I was fine, that I'd simply rolled my ankle.

Trevor was beyond upset when we returned. He couldn't understand why I'd put myself and the kids through such a crazy ordeal. In turn, I was furious at him. Didn't he understand I would never stop trying to live a normal life? I hated what was happening to me. There was no way I planned to let myself reach the point where I ended up like the lady at the bachelor auction, living in an aged care home surviving on puréed food.

I awoke each morning trying to convince myself that my life would be better than the day before. My positive outlook was generally quelled before breakfast finished. I was chronically sleep-deprived and constantly shouting at my kids. Then I'd torment myself with guilt for being a horrible parent. I felt like I was failing dismally at life. My son Jack often noticed how sad and angry I was. He'd look up at me with his sparkling blue eyes and say with sweet innocence, 'Please Mum, smile. When you smile, the whole world smiles with you.'

He'd grin at me until I did the same. Then he'd say, 'That's better!' and run off to terrorise his sister and wrestle his brother.

If only a smile could fix everything. I was being crushed slowly and inexorably by my situation. I eventually broke down, mentally and physically. Sadly, I hit the cold, hard ground of reality, and I conceded defeat. I began drowning in a deep well of depression. I felt numb, completely worthless. It was death by a million paper cuts. I turned to wine to ease my pain. I wasn't addicted to the alcohol per se, I was addicted to escaping reality. My self-destruction snowballed along with my self-loathing. My dis-ease with myself gave free rein to my harsh inner critic.

During this period, there were many times I once again toyed with the idea of ending my life. Only this time I knew there would be no rescue by a desperate, loving father pulling up in the family wagon. I figured I could drive into a tree and make it look like an accident because I couldn't bear the thought of leaving this world and having my kids think I'd given up on them.

I desperately needed to find a way out of my suffering, and soon, or I'd end up in a hole so dark and so deep that I'd never be able to climb out. So I called the suicide hotline. Yes, the girl who always vowed to soldier on regardless of the pain rang the 1-800 helpline. Since I was in a remote area, I was given a Skype appointment with a psychiatrist. He asked me a few questions and after four minutes prescribed antidepressants. I reluctantly agreed, but when one tiny pill left me nearly catatonic on the couch for a whole day I decided it was not for me.

I knew I wasn't depressed because of some hormonal imbalance in my brain. I was depressed because I believed my life sucked and I felt hopeless and powerless to change it. I didn't need medicating; I needed to see my situation differently. The problem was, I wasn't being grateful, I wasn't thinking about my husband's or my children's happiness. I was wholly focused on me and all the things going wrong in my life and totally ignoring all the other things that were going right. As they say, where the mind goes, the energy flows, and I was doing a stellar job of putting all of my energy into misery.

So often I've heard the advice, 'Do what you love, do what makes you happy.' For me, that meant leaving behind Jrudgerie, my family, my marriage, and what I perceived as my nightmare life to escape somewhere with palm trees and piña coladas. At the time I was reading *Eat, Pray, Love* and thinking, hell, if Elizabeth Gilbert could do it, why can't I? She found gelato in Italy, peace in India and a healer in Indonesia. Maybe if I found my own guru in Goa I could discover inner peace and then I'd be saved too.

In the meantime, I decided to do the next best thing and escape to Melbourne for the weekend. I was hoping to clear my head, maybe do some retail therapy and book into a masseuse to soothe my aching body. Anything to temporarily escape the pain of my tortured thoughts. And that's when I stumbled onto my salvation.

CHAPTER TWENTY-SEVEN
Wisdom from a Warrior Princess

Wherever you go, there you are.
~ Confucius

'I'm leaving my husband and children and moving to India after Christmas,' I announced in a muffled voice to the white tiled floor underneath me.

I sounded more like one of Alvin's Chipmunks than a severely depressed mother of three thanks to the fact I was lying face down on a massage table in Melbourne, my cheeks squeezed inside a padded hole. My lovely masseuse Michelle was listening to me ramble on about my life as she worked diligently on my aching back.

'Really? Why?' she asked, curiosity and concern etched into her voice.

'Because if I don't I'm as good as dead! I need to study Buddhism and change my perspective on life. I feel like it's the only thing left that can save me.'

It was the first time I'd used this particular massage therapist, and I found myself pouring my heart out to her. I felt like I was anonymous in Melbourne and could unload without fear of word getting out that I was dissolving into a mental mess. Just one of my many issues was that the drugs I'd been injecting every day weren't exactly working out well for me. My MS attacks continued unabated. My left leg could no longer lift on its own, and the simple act of walking now involved focused concentration. The only way I could step forward was by putting weight on my right leg and then swinging my left leg through, resulting in a pronounced limp and daily stumbles and falls.

I was angry and miserable about my situation and taking out my frustrations on all those closest to me. I should've known better, having read nearly every self-help book on the topic of self-sabotage.

'...and you know you don't have to go to India.'

What? My head popped out of the cushioned hole like a cork exploding from a bottle of champagne.

'Sorry, what'd you just say? I, uh, was a little distracted wallowing in my own self-pity,' I admitted sheepishly.

'I said, you don't have to go all the way to India to find Buddhism. They teach it here, upstairs, along with yoga.'

I couldn't believe what I was hearing. The universe had once again offered me a lifeline, a helping hand, just like the Czech hockey team in Italy and the job at the backpackers in Airlie Beach. For the first time ever I couldn't wait for a massage to finish so I could limp upstairs. The teacher who greeted me was a petite woman with a slick black bob and the chiselled features of a Maori warrior princess. She was tiny, fit and covered in tattoos from the neck down. She introduced herself as Sia. She was so far from the picturesque ideal of a serene, chubby Buddha-like guru, it was almost laughable. I felt as though I'd already been presented with my first lesson in Buddhist philosophy: 'Welcome to Preconceptions 101', better known as 'Don't Judge a Book by Its Cover'.

I was intimidated by Sia but also in total awe. She patiently explained the course had already started but that I could still join in. It was a blend of Buddhism, meditation and yoga that ran every Wednesday for four hours. I committed to a year of weekly classes, even though it meant an eight-hour round trip between Jrudgerie and Melbourne. I figured this was a far better option than flying to India. I walked out of the studio on a high, feeling like I was on the road to enlightenment.

My first class a week later was an eye-opener. I quickly realised the other students had been studying Buddhism for years and that whatever collective wisdom these people possessed was exactly what I was looking for. They were welcoming, kind, compassionate, calm and selfless. Above all, they seemed content. I felt like an imposter, much like the time I mingled with the rich and famous in my borrowed dress at the bachelor auction. This time however, the group was rich in happiness.

We began the class by sitting on the floor in a circle. Sia guided us through a meditation, asking us to focus on our breathing while she explained the virtues of *ahimsa*, practising non-violence towards other people and other living beings through our thoughts, words and deeds. This included being non-violent to ourselves as well. I wanted to cry when I heard this. I was my own worst enemy, a professional self-abuser who punished myself mercilessly for never being good enough.

'As you inhale, imagine a white light of love and peace entering into your heart. Allow yourself to feel lighter and happier, then, as you exhale, imagine sending a white light of love and peace to all beings as you say to yourself, "Let it go." Feel yourself being filled up with love, kindness and compassion and let any judgement or stress melt away.'

I breathed deeply, recited the 'let it go' meditation mantra in my head and immediately felt a weight lift off my heart. Even though we were only 15 minutes in, my anxiety and stress had eased. With the meditation complete, Sia launched into the concept of becoming a *bodhisattva*. She explained it was a Sanskrit word meaning 'enlightened mind'. Letting go of the ego, the self and cultivating compassion for all living things around you. Equal love without exception stemming from a desire to see all beings free from suffering.

The reason why everyone was so kind and content in the class was because, as Tibetan Buddhists, they were intentionally practising what is known as the six perfections—generosity, patience, moral discipline, joyful effort, meditation and wisdom—in order to take them further down the path to enlightenment. I loved the idea of it, but I figured I had to make a lot of changes in my life if I wanted to become a good Buddhist! I remembered my last stint in the school canteen when I had snuck extra ham on my kids' toasted sandwiches. If I was a good Buddhist I would have given every child extra ham! Well maybe not the Muslim boy, but I could've given him an extra falafel instead.

Sia continued with her lesson, oblivious to my conundrum.

'The biggest hurdle we face is overcoming our own suffering, because when we are unhappy we are in no condition to help others. And yes, it's a tricky balancing act. We need to look after ourselves so we can be content enough to stop worrying about our own happiness.'

I meekly put up my hand.

'Yes, Kat?' Sia looked at me with a raised eyebrow. 'And you don't have to put your hand up.'

The class laughed along with me as I let my arm drop to the floor.

'Um, I guess I'm a little confused. On the one hand you're saying, "Do what makes you happy," which for me usually involves getting a massage, drinking wine and eating chocolate. And on the other hand, you're saying this is selfish. Is making yourself happy a bad thing? I feel like it helps, at least for a while anyway.'

Sia replied carefully, 'Our true happiness is not derived from money or a massage or even chocolate! If Lindt balls were actually happiness pills, then every time you ate one your happiness would increase and the more balls you ate the happier you'd get, right? But that's not quite true, is it?'

It took me only a second to respond. 'Yes! When I eat too many I get a headache and then I feel guilty about devouring too many calories.'

'Exactly, so chocolate in itself doesn't create long-term happiness. The joy is fleeting and can eventually cause you pain. Money is the same. Every time you earn a dollar you aren't rewarded with a happy face emoji. You have to look beyond the external influences that temporarily satisfy your wants and desires to find real inner peace.'

She then quoted Śāntideva, one of the great Buddhist teachers.

'We are the authors of our own destiny, and being the authors, we are ultimately, perhaps frighteningly, free.'

It didn't take me long listening to Sia and the rest of the class to realise I was guilty of committing the mortal sin of continually recreating my own suffering. I'd become a constant complainer, spending most of the day ruminating about all the little things that irritated me, and the things I could no longer do. In fact, the karma of my selfishness was contributing to my depression, which I was trying to self-medicate with alcohol.

Noticing my discomfort, Sia asked gently but firmly, 'Kat, what do you really believe is the main cause of your suffering?'

I stopped and thought deeply about the question before replying as honestly as I could: 'I guess the root cause of my suffering centres around the fact I'm in constant pain with my back and I'm physically wasting away. MS has left me unable to do so many of the things I love to do. Simple acts like walking up the stairs to come to class today are challenging for me. The reality is, my future is bleak. I'm getting worse by the day. I try not to think about it, but the question is always there, lurking in my thoughts, how much time have I got before I have no quality of life left?'

The group listened silently and impartially to my words. No judgement here. I felt empowered.

'I constantly feel frustrated, angry and depressed. I feel trapped. I live in a desolate town in the middle of nowhere, my family is a million miles away in Canada. I have three kids who I love, but they never listen, and I constantly argue with my husband.'

I took a deep breath and spilled my deepest, darkest feelings.

'My Dad used to joke that I should have been drowned at birth. Maybe he was right. I've tried to be strong all my life, but now, and it kills me to admit it, I'm broken. If this is all there is to life, show me the exit sign. I want out.'

There were a few seconds of silence. The lady on my left, Maree, gave my hand a compassionate squeeze. I waited for someone—anyone—to tell me it was all going to be okay, that my 'woe is me' story was the worst they'd heard and that I was well within my rights to want to escape my situation. But Sia surprised me by holding a metaphysical mirror up to my face and reflecting everything I'd just said back at me.

'There's a famous Buddhist saying which states that all the happiness there is in this world comes from thinking about others, and all the suffering comes from a preoccupation with yourself.'

She stared directly into my eyes. 'My question for you is, why are you focusing on what you can't do instead of what you can do? You say you struggled to get to this class, yet here you are. You organised your family for the day, you drove your car here all the way from Jrudgerie and you climbed those stairs. You aren't broken. You need to stop beating yourself up. Remember, *ahimsa*, non-violence to yourself first.'

I nodded. The rest of the class gave me encouraging looks. No doubt, self-sabotage was nothing new to them and they were probably aware of its causes, unlike me. I was still living under the delusion that so many of my problems were someone else's fault.

'What you focus on and give energy to is what you will experience,' Sia noted. 'If you only think about your pain and what is hurting you, does that really help you feel better? You need to focus on the parts of you that aren't in pain. You need to start cultivating gratitude for the areas of your life that are going right. As for your husband and life in Jrudgerie, let me ask you something: who is looking after your kids while you are here? Your husband? If so, he obviously loves and cares about you enough to sacrifice his time to let you do this.'

Sia trailed off into silence, giving me time to digest her words. Spiritually, she was a lot like her physical persona, fierce and warrior-like. She tore off my self-pity like the layers of an onion, exposing my innermost misconceptions, selfishness and flawed worldview. Her words hit me with the force of a semi-trailer. I realised I needed to wake up to the story I was telling myself.

'All the reasons you are basing your suffering on, your need to escape, your anger, despair and frustration are creations of your own mind. You can't run away from yourself. Your suffering will follow, and while you may think you're trapped, the cage is of your own making. The key to successfully escaping is to change your perception of your situation. And you don't have to travel to India to do that.'

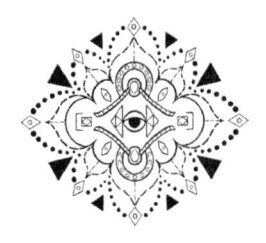

CHAPTER TWENTY-EIGHT
How Vegemite Changed My Life

The day I realised I could transform Vegemite into something I liked was the day I realised I could change everything I hated about my life.
~ Kat Finnerty

Slowly but surely, my weekly Buddhist classes began stripping away my preconceptions and exposing the real reasons behind my suffering. Namely, that I was my own worst enemy, too self-centred and angry at myself to see all the good surrounding me. I likened the process to a spiritual shaking by the scruff of the neck. It proved to be exactly what I needed. Sia was right. I didn't need to travel to India to find solutions to my problems. I needed to excavate the world within my head in order to dig out the truth. I'd created my own prison, and now it was up to me to break out of it.

During one class, Sia emphasised the importance of self-lessness, gratitude and perception as means of finding an end to suffering. She gave us a 'homework assignment' to complete over the week. We had to think about something simple that we hated and transform it into something we loved. I immediately thought of Vegemite. Yes, that vile, black yeast extract created after WWII in Australia to help baby-boomer mothers with nutrition. Trevor, like most Aussies, loved the stuff, but as far as I was concerned it was beyond disgusting.

There it was, my challenge for the week. Learn to love Vegemite sandwiches.

'We start small,' Sia explained, 'because if you can change your perception about Vegemite then you can change your perception about anything. It's going to be challenging, but,' she winked at me, 'you strike me as someone who enjoys a challenge!'

She was right. On the long drive to Jrudgerie I reflected on what I had learnt in class that day and needed to do. I felt transformed, rejuvenated, uplifted! I now realised I had a choice. I could begin to change my thinking or I could continue to blame the people around me, my illness and my past experiences for my anger, addictions and attitude. I needed to take responsibility for my life and focus on things that would promote peace, kindness and happiness.

When I pulled up to our little house in Jrudgerie, I was riding on a high and, for the first time in a long time, felt truly grateful for my simple surroundings. I was even grateful for the plate of overcooked veggies and chicken drumsticks Trev had prepared for my arrival.

I gave the kids a big hug, kissed Trev and sat down. They watched me curiously as I smiled and ate my dinner. Trev asked how the class had gone, and I explained about becoming a *bodhisattva* and about compassion and peace and love and Vegemite sandwiches and how lucky I was to have them all. My family were now looking at me with wide-eyed concern and wonder. Who was this crazy, blissed-out stranger?

'Well...okay then,' Trev said carefully. He put his plate in the sink. 'I guess that's good news. I know you've been struggling lately, so hopefully these classes will help get you back on track. We need this, Kat—*you* need this—'cause the way things were going...'

I nodded in agreement. 'Yes, I know, I know.'

Over the next few weeks I tried my best to meditate every day and follow my Buddhist teachings. I focused on what was going right in my world rather than what was going wrong, I tried to look at life as extraordinary rather than ordinary and sowed seeds of happiness whenever possible. I reminded myself, 'Before you act or speak, ask yourself, are you being kind?' For someone like me, who can be judgemental, prone to over-reacting and speaking without a filter, this turned out to be very hard to do.

I also decided to tackle my 'homework' by doing some research on how to make Vegemite delectable. I spoke to Vegemite lovers everywhere, asking them for hot tips, and was told the best way was to lather toasted white bread with butter and spread a thin veneer of Vegemite on top. I worked up the courage to diligently try this method over the next few days. And every time I did, I almost gagged. I tried mightily to convince myself the revolting taste in my mouth was actually delicious. But nothing seemed to change. It's all in your head, I'd tell myself. Taste is simply another perception you can change.

Finally, at the end of the first week, something shifted in my brain. Vegemite became bearable. It wasn't exactly the mouth-watering bliss I'd been instructed to turn it into, but it was now palatable. Progress! The exercise proved to be incredibly powerful, making me realise change was possible and that my perceptions could fundamentally alter my reality. Sia's words swam into my mind.

'Our thoughts are like the waves in the ocean. We can't stop the waves from coming, but we can choose which ones we want to surf.'

I tried the same technique on other foodstuffs formerly on my 'don't eat' list—olives, coriander, anchovies—and slowly began to transform my feelings about them as well. The lesson became clear. It was only my conditioning, past experiences and thinking that defined whether something was bad or good. Change your perception and—presto-chango—your world changes along with it. Of course, food was one thing; relationships and people were a whole different ball game. Although I did my best to alter my attitude and perceptions and spread the love to others around me, I only managed this with varying degrees of success.

One incident halfway through the second week perfectly outlined my struggle. I'd just finished doing the rounds of picking up the kids from school and kindy when Jack and Luke began tormenting each other in the back seat. I calmly asked them to stop and attempted to distract them with an 'I Spy' game. When that didn't work I tried Plan B, which was to take three deep breaths and think kind and loving thoughts to quell my rising anger. This was interrupted by Luke yelling at the top of his lungs, 'Stop it!' and violently kicking the back of my seat in response to Jack punching him in the shoulder.

I lost it. I screeched to a halt, turned around and screamed at the boys. The whole of Jrudgerie must have heard me. I immediately recognised my rookie error, and stopped mid-sentence. This was not doing anyone any good. With a supreme effort I calmed myself and assessed the situation for what it was. I thought, *What lesson can I learn from this?* Suddenly, the answer was obvious: Jack and Luke were simply mirroring my own behaviour! If I didn't want them to overreact and lash out when they were frustrated or angry, then I needed to act differently as well. I needed to build a longer fuse and stay in control.

And so it went. Applying my newly discovered Buddhist principles outside the classroom turned out to be difficult but worthwhile. Life was messy and challenging, and just because I'd decided to change didn't mean the universe had magically aligned itself to my beliefs overnight. It constantly threw circumstances and situations at me to test my resolve and willpower. I knew I was metaphorically slitting my karmic wrists every time

I became angry and lashed out, but it was as if I couldn't help myself. It was a vicious cycle of guilt and condemnation.

It took the Golden Rule of the Five Rs and the inspiring philosophy of a spiritual renegade in the form of a Harley-riding Buddhist monk to show me how to break out of my cycle of suffering and successfully fight back against my demons.

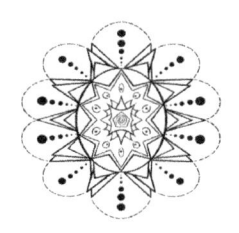

CHAPTER TWENTY-NINE
Planting the Seeds of Good Karma

Paddy says, 'Hey Mick, I'm thinking of buying a Labrador.'
'Are you crazy,' says Mick. 'Have you seen how many
of their owners go blind?'
~ Unknown

'I'm a failure, a fraud, a hypocrite,' I admitted morosely to my Buddhist class as they sat quietly around me, listening to my story.

'I constantly lose control and scream like a maniac at my kids, and then I'm so angry with myself that I secretly binge-eat crappy lollies, the same ones I've educated people for years not to eat. I follow it up with a bottle of wine. I poison and punish myself for my bad behaviour like some kind of deranged, self-abusing, candy-gorging, alcoholic psychopath. Then I feel so disgusted with my behaviour that I start the whole cycle again.'

Sia and the class nodded knowingly. I was spilling my guts out in an attempt to gain some much-needed help rather than elicit sympathy.

'Are you aware of the Five Rs?' Maree volunteered. In the last few weeks Maree had quickly become one of my favourite mentors in the class. She was warm-hearted, knowledgeable and compassionate, and I felt a deep connection with her.

I shook my head.

'They're a set of golden rules designed to help people when they screw up.'

She held up a closed fist and then listed each of the five Rs as she opened up her five fingers one by one.

'One—Recognise that I did or said the wrong thing.

Two—Regret that I shouldn't have done that.

Three—Recompense, how can I fix this or make up for it?

Four—Rejoice that I have now purified my mistake.

Five—Remember to do my best to not repeat it.

See? Now my hand has gone from closed to open. Your mind should be the same.'

I mulled over her wise words. Each rule was simple enough by itself. But when put together, the Five Rs created a powerful framework I could use to analyse and correct my mistakes while avoiding being consumed by guilt. They were a lifesaver. Finally, a process I could use to deal with the daily fails without beating myself up. I remembered what my yoga master Connor said:

'When you gain knowledge you gain wisdom. And if you then ignore that wisdom you are ignorant because you are ignoring the lessons learned.'

Sia tossed me a simple bangle. 'This is something small that will help keep you on the right track.'

I slipped it over my left wrist. She then challenged me to go 30 days without complaining about anything. Each time I complained either in my head or out loud I had to switch the bangle to a different wrist.

'Really? Do I have to?'

The group groaned and rolled their eyes. I cheekily changed the bangle to my right wrist. Okay, this was not going to be easy, but I was definitely up for the challenge.

'Keep this in mind, Kat. How people treat you is their karma; how you react to it is yours.'

And that's how we fell into our next topic of discussion; karma.

'Welcome to the Karma Café. There is no menu, you only get served what you deserve,' Sia announced with a laugh. She preempted the discussion by stating karma was perhaps the most widely misinterpreted concept in Buddhism. Like most people, I'd heard of karma, been told it was a bitch, but had no real understanding of what this actually meant. Some sort of cosmic payback scheme? I sat up and paid close attention when Sia began explaining how karma really worked.

'Karma is you with a GoPro strapped to your head. When you see yourself acting in kind, caring and loving ways, you invite love into your life. As a result, this is the movie you create. It's how your life will unfold. Conversely, if you see yourself blaming others for your problems or acting selfishly or in anger, you will attract the same. The movie you create for yourself will be about suffering. Karma has little to do with punishment or reward; it's simply the law of cause and effect, of reaping what you've sown.'

This went some way towards clarifying the concept for me. Karma wasn't really a bitch; it was more like a mirror! I thought about how I'd created both the good things in my life and, conversely, how I'd created all the mental pain I was now experiencing.

'Karma is about planting seeds, not about instant reciprocity,' Maree added. 'And when you plant those seeds, you need to do it from a position of love and kindness. The trick is not to expect something in return. We call this joyful effort with enlightened intention.'

Sia ended the class by adding, 'Remember, everyone, we don't have karma, we live karma. So if you want to change your karma and create a better future for yourself, you need to gift yourself a better story in the here and now.'

I returned to Jrudgerie with a new attitude and purpose. Amazingly, the following week I felt my perception of Jrudgerie shift in a hundred small ways. I realised the more I focused on being loving and kind, the kinder others were towards me. The more I reminded myself I was a calm and patient mother, the easier being a parent became. In comparison, the times I allowed myself to judge harshly, speak badly about someone or lose my cool with my kids or husband, I knew I was creating the conditions for the same thing to be thrown back at me. It also meant I had to constantly move my bangle from wrist to wrist!

This simple process helped me pay attention to how often I complained about the small things. It taught me to be more humble and less opinionated. Living in a small town, making assumptions about others' lives and then judging them for it is akin to a daily sport. It's easy to be sucked into the maelstrom, but when you realise it's also bringing you bad karma, it makes it much easier to opt-out.

At my next Buddhism class, I confided to Maree about my progress and she was over the moon for me. My anger and depression had receded dramatically, and my attitude towards life had fundamentally altered on so many levels.

'It's amazing! That karmic GoPro sitting on my head reminds me to approach situations and people in a more loving, kinder and gentler way,' I gushed excitedly. 'And having that awareness that things don't just happen, that it's all cause and effect, well…I feel like I'm more in control of my future.'

Maree nodded and smiled. I felt encouraged to go on.

'It's not easy. I have to monitor my thoughts like a hawk and I'm far from perfect, but I'm trying really hard.'

'Oh Kat, that's wonderful,' Maree replied. 'Perhaps you'd be interested in another teacher I've been following; he's got a really unique take on Buddhist philosophy. Have you heard of Lama Marut?'

I shook my head, intrigued.

Maree handed me a book titled *A Spiritual Renegade's Guide to the Good Life*. 'This man changed my life. Perhaps he will change yours too.'

I didn't take this statement lightly coming from Maree. Given how much had shifted in recent weeks, who knew what this book could do for me?

As soon as I returned home to Jrudgerie, I skimmed Lama Marut's biography. I was expecting a simple story about a monk's spiritual journey towards enlightenment but instead discovered the tumultuous life of a spiritual renegade. Marut was born into a strict Baptist family in Minnesota, and named Brian K. Smith. His father was a Baptist minister and as such, his childhood was steeped in religion. So it was no surprise when he went on to earn a PhD in comparative religion at the University of Chicago and became a professor of theology after teaching at Columbia University and the University of California. What was surprising was he also delved into the study of Hinduism and the ancient Vedic texts and even wrote a book about it. In his spare time, he pursued his passions for surfing, motorbike riding and long-distance running.

Paralleling his academic life was a turbulent private life littered with three marriages, three kids, an equal number of divorces and a mid-life crisis. He began suffering from chronic depression and anxiety that culminated in a complete mental breakdown, resulting in him being hospitalised and put on suicide watch. Soon after, he dropped out of academia and set out on a personal quest to find happiness. This quest eventually led him to Tibetan Buddhism, which radically changed his life.

After eight years of intensive study, during which he perfected the reading and writing of ancient Sanskrit, he was ordained as a monk and became known as Lama Marut.

Amazingly, when he was not touring the world with his assistant Cindy Lee, he was based in a remote part of Victoria here in Oz, not that far from my neck of the woods. I read more and found his story really resonated with the rebel inside me, especially the bit about why he considered himself a 'spiritual renegade'.

A spiritual renegade is someone who has had life kick their ass...who has had the rug pulled out from underneath them and wised up a bit, someone who has dropped the delusion that they have been singled out for suffering...and is willing to roll their sleeves up and do the hard work of making some inner changes so they can deal effectively with whatever life throws at them.

Wow! This was me in a nutshell. No wonder Maree had given me the book. I read and listened to everything I could get my hands on. His podcasts and teachings were unique, insightful, humourous and powerful. He didn't seem to care where the wisdom came from; Buddhism, Hinduism, Christianity, as long as they banished suffering and incited happiness. And then I stumbled onto something that would forever change the trajectory of my life. Lama Marut was conducting a retreat the following month at the Rocklyn Ashram near Daylesford, a four-hour drive from my doorstep. In outback terms, this was just around the corner. Here was my chance to learn from the legend in the flesh. There was no way in the world I was going to miss out on this opportunity! I likened myself to Princess Leia meeting Yoda for the first time, only my version was six-foot-plus, wore maroon robes and had far less hairy ears.

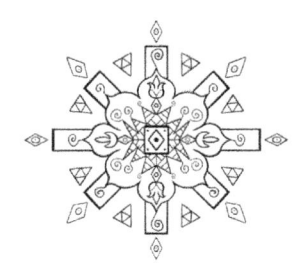

CHAPTER THIRTY
A Spiritual Renegade's Guide to the Good Life

'The spiritual quest is ultimately not the freedom of the individual; it is the freedom from the individual. And one of the main reasons we are not free is that the "somebody self" resists its own dethronement as the sole monarch ruling the Kingdom of Me.'
~ Lama Marut, Be Nobody

The rough, dusty road leading up to the ashram was lined by the majestic eucalypts of Wombat State Forest, which surrounded the facility on all sides. The buildings that emerged from the trees were functional and decidedly un-Indian looking, although they had a slight hippie feel thanks to their Hobbit-shaped windows and rendered mud-brick earthen walls. Families of kangaroos contentedly lounged on the grassy verge between the extensive gardens and the tranquil pond, diligently complying with the 'OM' symbol posted at the car park entrance.

My first impression was that this place was cocooned in its own bubble of peace, calm and contentment, somehow a part of but outside of the real world. As I walked in and presented myself to my fellow students, I was struck by how they all seemed to be trying to outdo each other in acts of kindness. It was endearing and slightly comical to observe.

After settling into the main meeting area on square cushions with the rest of the group, Lama Marut strode in with Cindy Lee by his side. He was a bear of a man, with a round face, close-cropped dark hair and kind eyes. His sleeveless maroon and gold Tibetan Buddhist robes only served to accentuate his size, but his mischievous smile radiated pure love. He welcomed us and then launched into an eye-opening lecture about what to expect from a 'guru'.

'A lot of people come to retreats like this thinking, now I've got a guru everything will be great. I'll have my own personal spiritual advisor on speed dial who can advise me on my most pressing problems. All I have to do is just listen and do whatever he says. But that's not how it works. Our job is to teach you the principles of how to live a happy life but it's up to you to do the hard work and apply them to your daily problems.'

He smiled and raised his eyebrows, as if challenging us to defy the logic. 'In fact, a lama or a guru is simply a divine sounding board, a mirror reflecting back at you what's good, what's bad, and what you need to fix, because ultimately it's all coming from you.'

Lama Marut then began comparing the lyrics of his favourite rock songs to some of the life lessons espoused by ancient Sanskrit sutras. He was humourous, intense and brimming with insightful wisdom.

And this is why I love this guy, I thought. His take on Buddhism may be quirky, but it's also powerful and relatable.

I turned my attention back to his talk. He was explaining how many people did not live with happiness as their main focus.

'…most of us, most of the time, are not prioritising the things that really matter — our personal spiritual training and self-discipline, and acts of kindness, altruism, and compassion toward others. We are instead consumed with, and diverted by, the very things that cause us more and more dissatisfaction.'

He insisted that the pursuit of true happiness was not a selfish desire but rather an altruistic one.

'I think one of the little demons inside our own heads that tries to trash our quest for true happiness is a wolf in sheep's clothing: "I thought you were supposed to be a good person who cared about others," that demon might say, "and here you are selfishly pursuing your own happiness." That's a devil that really needs a talking to, for the logic is totally faulty.'

Lama Marut tapped the table with his fingers and waggled his head to emphasise each point. 'We know from experience that it's only when we feel happy ourselves that we clear the head-space for taking real interest in others. We can't really be of much use to other people if we haven't fixed ourselves first.'

He was right. It was impossible to save the drowning, unless you knew how to swim. Lama Marut then reminded us that the goal of a spiritual life was not to be better than others but to be better for others. I nearly offered up an 'Amen!' but this wasn't a Baptist revival, and so I held back. Things became even more interesting when he began defining the secret to happiness.

'When we imagine what it's like to be happy, many of us picture ourselves living in this ecstatic state, like we're blissed out all the time. Now, I'm not sure that being blissed out all the time is possible or even desirable, but what's clear to me is that if we are to reach any of the higher states of happiness—joy, bliss, euphoria, ecstasy, or whatever—we must first achieve good ol' simple contentment.'

He glanced up and his eyes locked onto mine, as if he knew inherently I was struggling with this very concept. 'We're unhappy because we are dissatisfied with life and are driven by greed, aversion, grasping. As the Buddha said, *we suffer because we don't get what we want, we do get what we don't want, and we lose what we want to keep.* You wanna be happy and live more of the good life? Start with daily contentment and being grateful for what you have—that's what I like to call entry-level happiness.'

Of course! My chronic dissatisfaction with myself and others around me, including the place where I lived, was preventing me from leading a happy life. Here I was, trying desperately to mine precious nuggets of happiness out of each day and be the perfect mother and the perfect wife with the perfect body and perfect life, when all I needed to do was be content with who I was and what I had.

'What I'm offering you is a radical alternative to both fatalism, where you are perpetually feeling like a victim without agency, and a toothless spiritual stupor where just positive thinking is proffered as an effective method for making things better. This retreat is about taking the bull by the horns and providing you with the big ideas and powerful tools to change your life and create transformation.'

And he was true to his word. Over the next few days we learnt about perception and how to transform problems into opportunities, about how to free ourselves from fear and anxiety and unburden ourselves of past resentments. We created an action plan for obtaining true happiness. But by far my biggest revelation occurred over a lunch of chapatis and dhal while having a one-on-one chat with the man himself.

As I was recounting details of my disaster-prone life, Lama Marut stopped me mid-sentence and declared, 'Kat. Buddha wasn't kidding when he said life IS suffering. It's one of the four noble truths, along with the fact that suffering has a cause, it has an end and it has a cause to bring about its end.'

He stopped to dip his chapati in the daal. 'Remember, in this life, we're either in a disaster or between them. And without some kind of spiritual training we will always just be the victim of whatever new and improved calamity is waiting just around the corner.'

'But how do I avoid being a victim of my disasters?'

He answered with one of his trademark cheeky grins. 'Oh, that's easy. Just make sure to never let a good disaster go to waste.'

And with that he popped his chapati in his mouth and excused himself to discuss details of the afternoon session with Cindy.

I drove home to Jrudgerie a few days later feeling transformed. Perched on the passenger seat was precious cargo, a paper bag filled with a life-time's supply of tea towels, hand-embroidered with the life-changing words, *Never Let A Good Disaster Go To Waste*. A sticker on the outside of the bag espoused 'Happiness Tips' in brightly coloured letters.

Think less, feel more
Frown less, smile more
Talk less, listen more
Judge less, accept more
Complain less, appreciate more
Watch less, do more
Fear less, love more
POM - peace of mind

What made the tea-towels even more special was they had been created by my mentor Maree as part of her POM passion project, the proceeds of which went to a school in Sri Lanka.

My life was starting to feel like one great big Magic Eye drawing where suddenly I'd been shown how to pop out the secret image from the background chaos by looking at it from a different perspective. I felt like I was finally equipped with the right tools and superpowers to tackle my inner demons and address my most stubborn, persistent problems. I couldn't wait to unleash them on my world and see how my life would unfold.

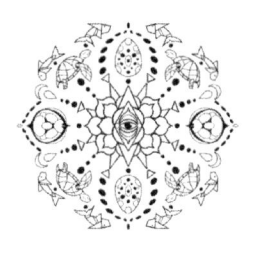

CHAPTER THIRTY-ONE
It's Like This Now

My happiness grows in direct proportion to my acceptance, and in inverse proportion to my expectations.
~ Michael J. Fox

I kicked off my crusade to create more of the 'good life' for myself with two powerful Lama Marut concepts: 'How to Make an Irritating Person Disappear' and 'It's Like This Now'. Irritating people are a part of everyone's lives. Sometimes the irritation is transitory, sometimes it's more deeply rooted. When I was a kid my number one irritating person was my younger brother. We had constant arguments. I used to complain to Dad, 'Martin is so annoying,' to which Dad would reply, 'Well, stop being annoyed by him!' Although this made perfect logical sense, I was eight years old at the time and had no idea how to do this!

In Jrudgerie, one of my biggest sources of irritation was the lady who ran the school canteen. She treated it as her own little fiefdom. She was demanding, miserable and controlling. But what irritated me most was her attitude towards healthy eating and nutrition. The canteen was a nuclear dumping ground for fast food and microwaved meals. Everywhere I looked there were frozen meat pies, sausage rolls and pizzas in plastic wrappers, as well as ice creams, chips and slushy machines. I'd long been an advocate of healthy eating, so when I volunteered to work in the canteen I made it my mission to introduce healthy, fresh food for the kids.

I decided to make her my Vegemite sandwich by transforming my utter disdain for her into understanding and love. It was going to be a big mouthful of ego to swallow. I skimmed over my notes from the retreat and listened to the suggested podcast entitled, 'How to make an irritating person disappear'.

Lama Marut's first words were, 'It's impossible to have an irritating person in your life unless you've been irritating yourself in the past. That's karma. And if you continue to be irritating back, all you're doing is perpetuating the cycle.'

Hmm, cause and effect. Wait a minute...that meant I was an irritating person too! I didn't think of myself as an irritating person, at least not like the woman in the canteen. I thought about my brother, father, husband, and kids. Okay, so maybe I could be considered annoying by some. Ouch, the truth hurts. Lama Marut went on to paraphrase Dad from all those years ago:

'Don't want an irritating person in your life? Stop being irritated by them!'

But he took the lesson a step further and gave me the spiritual knowledge to 'disappear' them.

'To stop the cycle, you can run away or stop talking to that person, but there's always another irritating person ready to fill the gap. Rather, you need to build up some spiritual muscles! When they start doing their irritating schtick, you just shut up and take it. Inside your head you might be thinking of all the four-letter words to describe that person. But nothing's coming out of your mouth. And then when you do speak, you give them back nothing but unconditional love. An irritating person is only irritating because you perceive them to be. For someone else they're not irritating at all!'

He also reiterated a lesson I'd learnt long ago in my army days—that often the person who challenges you the most in life turns out to be your best teacher.

I followed his advice. I didn't irritate the canteen lady in return. I practised patience and sent her love. Every time she annoyed me I told myself, *You're not perfect! You annoy other people too. What lesson can I learn from this? How can I cultivate compassion and love for her?* And soon the things that made her an irritating person in my mind slowly faded away until they disappeared altogether. Sure, the feeling may not have been mutual and we still didn't agree on food, but I was no longer creating bad karma for myself by being purposefully irritating and argumentative.

In essence, the irritating person turned out to be an analogy for every type of irritant in my life, not just the human kind. Every situation and event can be interpreted by us based on our likes and dislikes, our ingrained beliefs and attitudes. However, once you're aware of this, you can fundamentally change your perception and response. I discovered the irritating person concept worked equally well on small problems, like a cantankerous canteen boss, as it did on the larger ones, like children and a husband who sometimes drove me nuts. It was life-altering and allowed me to see the world through a whole different lens. Shakespeare summed it up perfectly: 'For there is nothing either good or bad, but thinking makes it so.'

With the success of the canteen lady notched on my trophy belt, I decided it was time to tackle my attitude towards Jrudgerie. I could not get my head around the fact that anyone could love the place when I disliked it so much. Again, Lama Marut came to my rescue. His philosophy of radical acceptance precisely encapsulated my situation. He explained how I could solve my problem in his typical renegade style.

Imagine there's a cosmic dealer handing out a set of cards to us every moment of every day. It doesn't matter whether we like the hand we are dealt; these are the cards we're allocated to play with. A skilful poker player will make the best of their cards, maximising the possibilities inherent in any situation. A bad poker player will fold too often, bet too much or try to bluff their way out.

In other words, he was urging me to live the best life I could within the reality of my present situation and to make the most of any new hand being dealt out.

Radical acceptance. Or in everyday parlance, it's like this now! Not 'It's like this now, but it shouldn't be like this' or 'It's like this now, but I wish it weren't like this' but 'It's like this now, and yes, even now.' Because radical acceptance wasn't just about accepting vanilla ice cream when no chocolate was available; it was about accepting the really crappy stuff too, the Vegemite-flavoured ice-cream, and responding in the wisest possible way.

So rather than complain about all the things I didn't like about my life, I began asking myself, 'Given it's like this now, what's the best way for me to respond for my present and future happiness?' And I realised that by acting from a *rational* rather than a *reactive* position, I could make much wiser choices about how I thought about my life and what actions I needed to take to ensure a better future.

To my amazement, my new attitude started paying off almost immediately. I began to feel like I belonged. I stopped pretending to be outwardly happy and concentrated on becoming more inwardly content. I cast off my mantle of victimhood and started planning a way out of my predicament. This included renewing my efforts to pursue a path of healing and a possible cure for my MS, even though I knew this path would be littered with hardship, uncertainty and pain. But my mindset had been buoyed and uplifted by Lama Marut's wise words and my courage and conviction was now fortified by a tried and tested 2,500-year-old philosophy designed to transform suffering. The timing could not have been better and the stakes could not have been higher. The biggest battle of my life lay ahead of me.

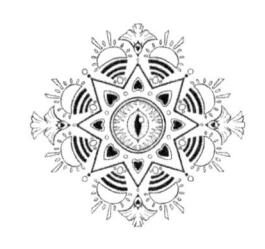

CHAPTER THIRTY-TWO
The MS Roller Coaster

What's the difference between a doctor and God?
God doesn't walk around thinking he's a doctor.
~ Dr Czemy, Chicago Med

Living with MS was like playing a never-ending game of Russian roulette. Occasionally, there were blanks in the chamber, but live rounds were always imminent, and when the bullets started firing things became very real, very quickly.

I suffered countless attacks, most of them exacerbated by stress. With three kids in three years, just being alive was stressful! Attacks would sneak up and hammer different areas of my body, depending on which part of my brain or spinal cord was affected. At different stages during my life I lost the use of my right arm, my left arm, my left leg, my bladder and the vision in my left eye. I suffered fatigue, nerve pain, pins and needles and muscle spasms.

Each time I was attacked I fought back with a solid dose of intravenous steroids. It was a relief when I was able to use the limb again, even though it would never quite work the same. In the back of my mind, I always knew the next attack could leave me permanently disabled. I did my best not to allow myself to think that way. Rather, I put my time and energy into finding alternatives, knowing attacks and eventual disability were inevitable if I were to rely solely on what modern medicine prescribed.

For a start I devised a holistic approach to my healing, adopting a therapeutic diet, experimenting with supplements and meditating regularly. I left no stone unturned in my quest to avoid ending up in a nursing home. I went to naturopaths, psychics, doctors, and faith healers—as an aside, I now know why you fall backwards when you're struck by the healing power of God through a faith healer's hand because they hit your forehead pretty bloody hard—and it was all helping, it just wasn't a cure.

The psychic I visited announced I would heal myself but was vague about how. However, she did inform me I would leave my husband and find true love with a tall, dark-haired man on a remote tropical island, which was kind of interesting. I would know it was the right man apparently, because a sapphire was involved. I dismissed this bizarre statement out of hand. I was looking for a cure for my health issues, not a prophecy about my love life. The naturopaths were a little more specific. I was told to eliminate all inflammatory and acidic foods—no sugar, wheat, dairy, or meat. I lived for years on sprouted mung beans, vegetables and fish. The radical change of diet may not have cured all the damage I'd already sustained, but it did dramatically lessen the number of subsequent attacks and gave me a sense of being in control of a somewhat uncontrollable disease.

I took a dose of incredibly expensive bovine colostrum made from specially bred New Zealand cows that—based on the cost of the colostrum—may or may not have lived in luxury stalls with hot and cold running water. It didn't work. I tried acupuncture and magnetic therapy. I even had electrodes attached to my head and feet to send pulses of electricity through my body at a certain vibrational frequency while I was bathed in healing, coloured lights. None of it worked.

I gave low-dose naltrexone (LDN) a whirl. This is a drug given to alcoholics and heroin addicts, albeit at ten times the strength, to stop them from spiralling into depression after a high. LDN floods the brain with endorphins, which helps reduce inflammation throughout the body, the root cause of MS. The therapy worked, at least to the extent it halted and almost eliminated the symptoms of one of my attacks. But it still wasn't a viable option to stop my long-term deterioration.

I was constantly slapping a Dr Ho's TENS machine on different parts of my body and cranking up the electrical current through the sticky pads, hoping it would stimulate my damaged nerves and revive my weakened muscles or counteract muscle spasms. Sometimes I'd become super ambitious and turn the machine to max, causing my limbs to flail around wildly. There was one particular time I had a Dr Ho's shoved down my pants while I was driving. I was trying to stimulate my hip flexor and adductor muscles. Momentarily distracted, I realised too late that the car ahead of me had braked for some reason and the next thing I knew I was surrounded by smoke, my airbags had gone off and a passerby was banging on my window asking me if I was all right. The accident was less about Dr Ho affecting my leg control and more about me not paying attention, but it took me a long, long time to explain what I had down my pants and why to the cops that showed up a short time later.

I investigated worm therapy, thought to dampen the body's immune response. It was promoted by an alternative American medical practitioner who deliberately gave himself worms sourced by walking through the cesspools of Calcutta. For a small fee he'd send you his excreted worms by post. I contemplated this for a while but decided that deliberately ingesting someone else's faecal worms was best kept in the 'last resort' box.

I looked into bee sting therapy, in which a sadistic naturopath would sting you with 20 to 40 bees on different parts of your body in order to create inflammation. The body would then mount an anti-inflammatory response, resulting in reduced inflammation in other parts of the body. Possibly good for the patient, but not so good for the bees. I couldn't find enough convincing evidence to be the murderer of hundreds of honey makers and pollinators or, more to the point, endure dozens of tiny little bee needles entering my flesh.

I gave tremor therapy and vibration machines a red-hot go. Tremor therapy involves loading your limbs with weights and moving super slowly until you shake under the strain, then repeat ad nauseum. It's supposed to recalibrate and stimulate the nervous system, just like the vibration machine. I tried them both but noticed very little difference, perhaps because I wasn't committed enough. I still believe they have some merit, however, and continue to occasionally use them therapeutically.

I researched chronic cerebrospinal venous insufficiency, less cumbersomely known as CCSVI. A doctor in Italy by the name of Zamboni claimed he had cured his wife's MS by radically increasing the blood flow from her brain to her heart. I thought this had potential and did some serious digging into the topic. Eventually, I would go ahead with this procedure, but not with Dr Zamboni and not until my 40th birthday many years later.

Suffice to say, the result of all this stone turning was...a giant pile of stones! I became an expert on all possible cures. Trying out alternative therapies wasn't an act of desperation—okay, maybe a little—but had more to do with my innate character and my newly acquired mindset. I refused to give up. Go hard or die trying was me in a nutshell.

So you can only imagine my euphoria when I discovered a radical new therapy for MS being offered by a clinic in Israel involving stem cells that promised not just the potential for remission but also the reversal of some or all of my symptoms. Could this possibly be the miracle I'd been looking for?

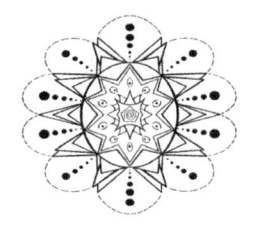

CHAPTER THIRTY-THREE
Salvation in the Promised Land

*Our lives are fashioned by our choices. First we make our choices.
Then our choices make us.*
~ Anne Frank

It was 2007, and the rumours surrounding stem cells and their ability to cure a variety of incurable diseases even managed to reach me in Jrudgerie. Stories were swirling around the media and the medical fraternity like a mini-tornado. My first attempt to research stem cell therapy on Dr Google wasn't exactly encouraging. *Stem Cell Therapy: Miracle Cure or Dangerous Experiment? 21st Century Snake Oil—Promise Vs Reality.* It seemed the mainstream medical establishment was split down the middle on the treatment: some thought it would revolutionise modern medicine while others thought it was highly dubious, saying it over-promised and under-delivered.

Within MS circles, the hype was around mesenchymal stem cells, MSCs, which seemed to combat inflammation in the body by regulating the immune system. It was claimed MSCs had the potential to halt the progression of MS and repair some of the damage already done. If so, this was nothing like the disease-modifying drugs currently being offered to me as a treatment plan, because they only moderately helped slow the progression of the disease. This treatment had the potential to be a game-changer of epic proportions.

The clincher for me was my dad told me about our neighbour Louise. She was an up-and-coming pro golfer, who was diagnosed with primary progressive MS just as she was making a name for herself. Hers was a far more aggressive version of MS than mine. Within months, the disease left her struggling to walk. Her neurologist, aware of the dire nature of Louise's situation, knew there was little that could be done for her in Canada, so he directed her to a cutting-edge clinic in Israel. She ended up being one of the first adult stem cell therapy recipients at the Weizmann Center. And it worked! She was back to making par in no time.

After a long distance call with Louise and comparing the alternatives, I decided this was my best chance for a cure. There was only one small stumbling block. The treatment was going to cost more than $40,000, a small fortune for me. I mentioned this to a friend in Jrudgerie, noting that while I believed the procedure might save me, it would take some time to gather together such a huge sum of money. A few weeks later I opened my front door to find a news crew on my doorstep. Amy, the reporter, explained she wanted to capture my reaction regarding the community's fundraising efforts for my procedure.

'Fundraising? For me?' And this was when I first heard about the communities of Jrudgerie and surrounds secretly banding together to raise nearly $12,000 for my stem cell treatment. I was flabbergasted! Amy informed me that a core group of my friends, along with Trevor's family, had sent countless letters summarising my story and asking for donations. And now, together with the mayor and the rest of the town, they were planning a big function at the local golf club where I would be the guest of honour and would be invited to speak about my hopes for a cure. The local paper was on board to report the good news and document my journey.

Thanks to the media attention and the hard work of my friends and family, hundreds rallied to support my cause. Around $20,000 was raised, an incredible achievement considering the tiny size of our community and the fact the district was going through a severe drought at the time. It thoroughly demonstrated the generosity of the community's spirit. The situation was surreal, inspiring and humbling. Who would have imagined that the town I never wanted to call home, where I'd always felt like an outsider, would band together to help me? How could I have been so blind?

I became a sort of mini-celebrity overnight. In addition to the local TV and regional newspapers running stories on me, I was featured in *The Australian Jewish News* thanks to my connection to Judaism through my mother. The Jewish National Fund contacted me to offer a donation of money and asked if I wanted to celebrate this life event by planting a tree on a mountainside near Jerusalem. Boy, did I ever.

In the meantime, my family and friends in Canada had also begun organising a fundraising campaign: a golf day followed by a dinner and silent auction at a country club. They called it 'Kat's Kause'. It too was a sold-out event with more than a hundred people in attendance. Another $20,000 was raised.

Within a month of deciding to go ahead with the therapy the entire cost of the procedure was covered, not only by people who loved and cared about me but also by generous strangers who just wanted to help. All the seeds of love and kindness I'd been planting had seemingly ripened. If that's not karma, I don't know what is.

It was at this stage the clinic in Israel contacted me. They required a thorough examination and a recent MRI scan. So off I went to see my current neurologist to obtain the required paperwork. Dr Alphabet had sadly moved on years earlier. My new neurologist was tall, middle-aged and studious and wore wireframe glasses. He was polite enough but brandished his intelligence like a sword, wielding it impatiently whenever I questioned him about alternatives to the drugs he prescribed. He radiated superiority. I felt more than a little intimidated by him.

He began his examination by having me lie on my back and asking me to lift one leg at a time and press it as hard as I could against his hand. I was completely unable to move my left leg. He made some notes and went through a few more tests before asking me to stand and walk heel to toe. I couldn't. He then instructed me to balance on one leg, which I tried valiantly to do, but I had to hold his arm to stop myself from falling. My balance was non-existent.

'What medication do you take currently?' he inquired.

I replied, 'A strict therapeutic diet, exercise, meditation, and sunlight.'

'No, no,' he waved his hand impatiently. 'Which disease-modifying drug are you on?'

'None,' I said. 'I've tried several of the MS injections, but none of them have really worked, and the needles are literally a pain in the ass. I've been managing with natural alternatives. But now I'm going to Israel for stem cell treatment. All I need is a referral letter and an MRI please.'

He looked at me as if I'd just told him I was going to cure myself by scattering rose petals around my bed while saying the alphabet backwards. He remarked, rather haughtily, that the concept was interesting, but from what he'd heard, it didn't work.

'It's experimental, and there are major risks, but it's your choice. From my point of view you'd be better off sticking to the tested MS medications on the market. I'll try to keep an open mind given you seem determined to go through with this,' he remarked somewhat scornfully.

An open mind...yeah, right!

Trevor came with me to Israel for the first part of the treatment, which involved a bone marrow aspiration. I met my doctors, Dr Slavin and Dr Gesundheit, at the Weizmann Center. They were professional, patient and kind, and I felt blessed to know both of them. Dr Slavin stuck a giant needle more suitable for a horse than a human into my hip. Luckily, I was knocked out for this procedure.

The goal was to harvest the MSCs in my bone marrow, which were unique because they could turn into every other cell type in my body. Once removed these cells were transferred to a specially designed clean room in order to culture them for about four weeks until they multiplied exponentially. The microbiology lab would then test the new cells to confirm sterility. Getting the last part right was crucial because any contaminated cells, if injected back into me, could be fatal.

Both doctors were very clear about the risks I was taking. They admitted the procedure was still in its infancy and highly experimental, but the chance of a full recovery was possible. They noted that as I was opting not to do chemotherapy before the transplant, it was likely I'd need a booster shot within a few years. Bonus! The booster would be half-price. They would freeze some of my MSCs so I wouldn't have to endure another horse needle in the hip. Thank God for small mercies.

Remarkably, the final part of the therapy, in which the sterile fluid is injected into your spine, could not be performed in Israel.

'According to Israeli law,' explained Dr Gesundheit, 'we are able to take things out of you but not put anything in. We will send you to a hospital in either Greece or Turkey when your cells are ready.'

God bless him.

Straight after the bone marrow aspiration in Tel Aviv, Trev and I were picked up by a representative of the Jewish National Fund, along with a reporter and cameraman. They whisked us away to a mountain overlooking Jerusalem. I planted my tree amongst a grove of thousands, each planted by people like me who had a connection to Israel and then read a moving poem. I was now leaving two pieces of myself in Israel, one in a lab and the other in the shape of a living tree, both symbols of hope and optimism for a better future.

Six weeks later my cultured cells were ready and I received the call to go to Greece. Trevor stayed home to look after the kids, so I was accompanied by my childhood friend Jenn and her extended family. They'd flown all the way from Canada to support me.

The day of my procedure happened to coincide with my 35th birthday. I'll never forget arriving at the hospital with Jenn. It was filthy and filled with people smoking in the corridors. Seriously, this was the place my Israeli doctors had chosen for me to have my sterile MSCs injected into my spinal cord?

I found my room and met my roommate, a woman named Kelly. She was also from Canada and, like me, had three kids, was a nutritionist and a runner and had MS. It was like meeting my doppelgänger. A representative from the Weizmann Center flew in, delivered the vials of our harvested cells to our bedside and disappeared. Soon after, a woman in a white coat, who I assumed to be a doctor, strode in. She spoke little English and was quite abrupt. For some unknown reason, she seemed irritated by having to perform the procedure on us.

The process, as explained to us in Israel, involved inserting a needle into our spines to withdraw a precise amount of cerebrospinal fluid, which would then be replaced with the same amount of fluid containing the harvested cells. I'd undergone spinal taps in Melbourne, and the procedure was always performed under sterile conditions. Here in Athens, the doctor didn't even wash her hands in between injecting Kelly and then turning around to my bed to do me.

I did my best to banish any fearful thoughts, instead replacing them with those designed to bring me good feelings. I envisioned celebrating my birthday at dinner that evening in a fine Greek restaurant, eating the best moussaka and baklava and sculling shots of eye-watering ouzo, in a toast to the start of my new life.

As instructed, I curled into a ball and exposed my spine. Jenn held my hand. My eyes were squeezed tight. The woman jabbed the needle into my back. She cursed in Greek and yanked it out. I felt the needle again being plunged into my back. I flinched from the pain and counted down from three to calm myself. Meanwhile, the doctor's mobile started ringing with the ringtone of the Rolling Stones' 'I Can't Get No Satisfaction'. She cursed impatiently and again withdrew the needle.

On the third jab I heard and felt something inside me go 'snap'. It reverberated through my body like a gunshot. I screamed and my eyes flew open. I dug my nails into Jenn's hand.

Breathless, and through gritted teeth, I said, 'She's hit something.'

The doctor, in her heavily accented English, barked out, 'Wat? Wat?' But I waved her off and indicated that I was okay. I calmed my breathing, closed my eyes and curled into a tighter ball. This was no time to be faced with a needle-wielding doctor and a language barrier.

Finally, on the fourth attempt, the doctor successfully penetrated my spinal cord, removed a couple of CCs of spinal fluid and replaced it with the harvested cells. In Israel, Dr Slavin explained that after the injection, we would have to lie on our backs with our feet elevated at the head of the bed so the new stem cells could migrate down to our brains. This is exactly what Kelly and I did. The Greek doctor let us know that we were to stay still for the rest of the day and then we could leave. I would be able to celebrate my birthday with an authentic Greek dinner.

I encouraged Jenn to take off for a few hours and enjoy exploring Athens with her family. In between, I would meditate, read and relax for the remainder of the day. Neither of us realised the hell that would shortly be unleashed.

I'd been reading for about half an hour when Kelly began groaning. She was massaging her temples, complaining her head was pounding. The emergency buzzer to summon help was at our feet, just out of reach. I screamed for the nurse and threw my book at the door. Kelly was rapidly deteriorating, crying and writhing in agony. Despite being warned not to move, she dragged herself up and hit the help button. Moments later, whatever was happening to Kelly slammed into me like a wrecking ball.

The pain was excruciating. It felt like someone was smashing a hammer relentlessly against the inside of my skull. This was far beyond any migraine pain I'd endured as a child; it was even worse than giving birth. I didn't scream or cry out. I lay motionless and silent, gritting my teeth. I resorted to doing what I always did when I experienced severe pain: I detached from it. I prayed for something I normally dreaded: a needle—preferably one full of morphine!

We theorised later that the incompetent Greek 'doctor' with the shocking bedside manner had probably injected too much of the fluid containing our harvested stem cells into our spinal cords, causing the pressure to build up and our brains to swell. The next four days were a blur of intense, excruciating pain as I slipped in and out of consciousness. Having an experimental medical procedure go terribly wrong was the ultimate test for practising radical acceptance. This was ten levels above accepting boring old vanilla in place of chocolate ice cream. I reminded myself to take responsibility for my reactions, even if I wasn't responsible for the situation. *Come on Kat! Give your brain a chance to step out of that feedback loop of pain and fear and breathe calming, healing breaths.*

At one stage I recall Kelly pacing the room, half-naked and crying. Every now and then a nurse would come in and give us a shot of pain relief, but it hardly took the edge off. I ate and drank nothing. Jenn and her family did their best to help, but there was little they could do. Whenever my situation threatened to overwhelm me, I prayed to God for help and offered up my suffering. I decided to try and 'let go and let God'. Dad would have approved. It's funny how, when faced with our own mortality, our faith is suddenly resurrected like Jesus at Easter. I used everything I had in my arsenal to make it through the subsequent days: Connor's Connorisms, Lama Marut's meditations and my dad's pragmatic approach to pain.

In the meantime, the hospital staff made it very clear they wanted us out. The one-day procedure that Israel had paid for had turned into four yet-to-be-paid-for days of hell. The administration insisted we had to leave. At this stage, I had no idea whether the stem cell therapy had worked or not. I didn't even know if I could walk. Jenn and her mother tried to sit me up, but I collapsed back as soon as they let me go. It was obvious there was something wrong with my back. This was why I hadn't been able to move over the last four days. The penny dropped.

'Jenn,' I whispered, 'I...I think I'm partially paralysed.'

Jenn began screaming at the doctor and nurses standing at the foot of my bed. 'What have you done? What have you done to them?'

I glanced at Kelly. She was rocking back and forth, curled in a ball, crying and saying she couldn't handle the pain anymore. Amidst the chaos, I focused on the mantra, 'This too shall pass. This too shall pass. This...too...shall...pass.'

With a supreme amount of effort, I forced myself to stay calm. But there was no denying something had gone horribly wrong. A voice deep in my mind was whispering, 'Oh God, Kat, what have you done?'

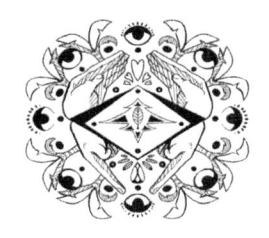

CHAPTER THIRTY-FOUR
The Road to Recovery

*I judge you unfortunate because
you have never lived through misfortune.
You have passed through life without an opponent—
no one can ever know what you are capable of, not even you.
~ Seneca*

Paralysis is a strange affliction. It's essentially the absence rather than the addition of something. People can catch a cold, sustain an injury, develop cancer or display symptoms of disease, but when you're paralysed you lose feeling, you lose motion, you lose a piece of yourself. It's scary, frustrating, demoralising, and debilitating.

Contracting MS meant I was used to losing pieces of myself, but this time the situation was different. I couldn't fix my back with a big dose of steroids. I didn't know if it could be fixed at all. I was in unknown territory. As Jenn and her mother tried to get me to stand, I discovered I could no longer bend at the waist. I had almost no forward flexion. I was unable to dress myself, couldn't put on my shoes or even my undies.

I took a few deep breaths. If Lama Marut was here, he'd remind you to avoid attaching to bad outcomes, the *what ifs*, and instead concentrate on what you can do right now, in this moment, to create a better story.

And there was some good news. I could actually stand upright with some help, although when I walked I looked like a tiny Frankenstein monster, stiff from the waist up. Best of all, after taking a few tentative steps, I cottoned on to the fact my left leg seemed to be working almost normally. No longer did I have to swing it forward. I could lift it and put one foot in front of the other without conscious effort.

Sweet Jesus, maybe the therapy worked!

I managed to stagger out of the hospital under my own steam and spent the next few days convalescing in a holiday house Jenn's family had rented before flying back to Canada and into the welcoming arms of my family. Sadly, I never did manage to blow out the flame on a celebratory birthday ouzo shot because my brain was still pulsating in my skull, but I did enjoy a wonderful meal of moussaka and baklava before I left Greece.

My dad and my siblings were very concerned when they saw the state of me a week after the transfusion. At this stage, my inability to bend hadn't changed. I struggled to get in and out of the car, I still couldn't put on my own underwear and I had to do some interesting manoeuvres just to rise up out of bed. My left leg continued to work on its own however, and the numbness and pins and needles down the entire left side of my body were fast becoming a distant memory. I was equally elated and troubled. The procedure seemed to have worked, but at what price?

I went to our family doctor to see if he had any idea how to fix me or what might be going on. I filled him in on my journey and experiences in Greece, including the loud snap I'd heard and felt when the doctor jabbed me in the spine.

He rubbed his chin and postulated, 'It's most likely she hit a nerve. There is no telling at this stage if the damage is temporary or permanent, only time will tell. Seriously Kat, what the hell were you thinking, taking a risk like this? Medical tourism for experimental procedures is foolish. It kills people. There is a reason we have laws about what we can and cannot do to people in this country.'

His lecture infuriated me. Foolish? From my perspective, it would have been foolish to watch my life slip away and end up in a nursing home. I'd always known there were risks associated with the procedure, but the risks were well worth it when compared to the alternative. I shuffled out of the doctor's office, determined to heal myself.

It was time to figure out the purpose hidden within my pain and discomfort. I didn't believe it had anything to do with stoically enduring the suffering and complications arising from my operation. Rather, it had to do with the way I looked at my overall situation. Maybe the lesson was about patience and gratitude. Maybe it was yet another reminder about the universal nature of suffering; that unwanted things happen all the time and ultimately it was up to me to choose my response. What was it Epictetus said? 'Disease is an impediment to the body but not to the will, unless the will itself chooses.' Considering I'd only just returned from Greece, the birthplace of Stoicism, and that Epictetus was one of its foremost thinkers and scholars, I figured it might be wise to take on some of his advice.

I thought a little more about how a true Stoic would view my situation. There was no doubt they'd see it as an opportunity to respond with virtue, courage and strength, a chance to build up character and wisdom. They'd point out that life is always unpredictable and throws perils and impediments our way and that this can ultimately be freeing if we view it as a challenge to be embraced. So that's what I did.

Over the next few weeks I began an intensive regime of yoga, acupuncture, gym work, massage, and chiros. I made it my quest to bend and walk normally again. My sister even dragged me along to her Zumba class where I did a fair-to-middling impression of a zombie from Michael Jackson's 'Thriller' video.

Each day I made incremental improvements and repeated the same mantra: 'Never, never, never give up'. Day after day I exercised and stretched for hours. I visualised and manifested being able to bend and walk normally, to balance on one leg and, when I allowed my imagination to really go wild...I even dreamed about running. And what I discovered was that through persistent effort, change is possible when accompanied by a passionate belief. The fact that daily changes were minuscule mattered not. I was moving forward, not backward.

A month later I returned to Australia. When I spotted Trevor and the kids waiting at the airport with a sign, 'The Donovans from Jrudgerie', I dropped my bags and ran towards them. It was the first time my five-year-old daughter had ever seen me run, let alone walk without a pronounced limp. They were deliriously happy to see me. Trev was in tears, amazed that both my back and my legs seemed to be cured. So was I.

In the ensuing weeks Kelly and I put a complaint forward about our treatment in Athens, and as a result, no patients were ever treated there again. The ABC's '7:30 Report' tracked me down and interviewed me at their studio in Sydney. It was big news. I had reversed years of disability by using stem cell therapy, and so had another Australian, a boy named Ben who lived in Canberra.

I desperately hoped our stories would be the beginning of a revolution in the treatment of MS and would inspire others to be courageous enough to defy the status quo of Big Pharma. You can only imagine my excitement when I finally got the chance to show off my improvement to my sceptical neurologist two months after the transplant. I imagined how stunned and speechless he would be when I showed him I could run again. The implications were huge for all his other MS patients. This was the cure everyone was waiting for. I was walking, talking, running proof that stem cell transplantation worked!

I could barely contain myself when I walked into his office. When he asked me to lift my leg, I raised it without effort.

When he asked me to walk heel to toe, I smashed it—not even a teeter. I could even balance on one leg and do a twirl. By the time we finished, I was bursting with pride. I'd accomplished every test with flying colours.

The doctor motioned for me to have a seat while he compared the notes of my previous examination to my current one. I had to sit on my hands to stop myself from clapping with glee. He sat shaking his head, then looked over his glasses at me, and stated, 'Your condition has not changed, in fact, your strength is declining. You need to stop being so foolish and reckless and go back on the MS medication.'

I was dumbstruck. Surely he was joking.

'How exactly did you arrive at that conclusion?'

'Well, you see, the pressure of your leg against my hand when I asked you to lift it wasn't as strong as at your previous consultation.'

I was perplexed. At my previous consultation I couldn't lift my leg at all. Let alone balance on one foot. His 'conclusion' was completely subjective and based on a misguided belief in his own superiority, knowledge and authority. The medical books, the drug companies, they all claimed stem cell therapy for MS didn't work, and so that was the story he'd decided to believe, despite being presented with overwhelming evidence to the contrary.

I don't think he had any idea how soul-destroying his words were or how they affected me. I wanted to scream, 'How dare you?!' at the top of my lungs. Not only was he discrediting my treatment and all my efforts to make myself whole again, but he was also denying other MS patients the opportunity to see what a life without disability and disease looked like. Sure, there was a risk that the stem cell therapy would not last forever and may require booster infusions, but it was far better than any of the alternatives on offer so far. And even though in my heart and soul I knew the stem cell therapy had made my body better, not worse, I still allowed him to plant a seed of doubt in my mind. Perhaps this contributed to the fact that not long after, I inexplicably lost the ability to run.

Over the next few years I tried my best not to allow my neurologist's negative prognosis to further infiltrate into my thoughts and affect my life. I'd done too much work on healing my mind and body to fall down that well of despair again. I was now a hell of a lot more mobile. I didn't dread stairs, I didn't struggle to lift my leg into the car and I was not stumbling or falling nearly as much as I used to. As the years passed without even a hint of a relapse, I saw no need to go back on a regime of MS drugs. Also, I had my Plan B: the MSCs frozen in a lab in Israel.

I threw myself into life with as much joyful effort, contentment and gratitude as I could muster. Sure, there were still hiccups and stumbles, but these situations were the exception rather than the rule. My fitness business was doing really well, mostly because I loved what I did. The only drawback was I worked opposite hours to Trev. I'd be gone early morning and evenings, and he'd work all day and arrive home just as I was leaving again. We became expert tag-teamers, working around a never-ending stream of commitments to work, horse riding, school events, sport competitions and training sessions. We hardly spent any time together. And when we did we were usually either catching up with jobs that needed doing at home or too tired and distracted to have a half-intelligent conversation.

Search and Destroy kept us busy with their footy and cricket, while Stella diverted my spare time into the world of horses. I even got to run the Pony Club canteen and create my own fiefdom of healthy deliciousness. I know, karma right? What wonderful stuff!

Trev was supportive of my dedication to the world of horses, Buddhism, fitness classes, yoga retreats, and yearly trips home to Canada. However, he did find the constant jet-setting mildly manic.

'Why can't you just relax, be content with how things are here in Jrudgerie?' he'd question in his chilled-out, easy-going way.

He wasn't wrong. I just felt like I needed new ways to challenge and better myself every day. I wanted to make a difference in the world. I was committed to living a life of purpose. Trev, ever the optimist, saw the beauty and potential in Jrudgerie and was keen to get into the house-flipping game. Partly to placate him and partly to spend more time together, we began attending courses on real estate and investment. We quickly learned Jrudgerie's downside also had an upside. Unlike other more popular towns in the region, houses in Jrudgerie were dirt cheap to buy.

We hatched a plan to begin buying dumps for a cheap price, fixing them up to rent out and eventually sell. I was hoping this would give Trev and I the financial freedom and independence to pack up the family and leave Jrudgerie once and for all.

Some weeks later I was contacted by a lady whose daughter was relocating to Jrudgerie for work. She wanted to buy some fitness sessions for her as a moving gift. She also enquired if I knew of any nice places for rent. Not surprisingly, her daughter was having a hard time finding anything decent to live in. It just so happened there was a property Trev and I were thinking about buying that had been on the market for years but needed a few weeks of renovation work to bring it up to scratch. We put in a good offer with a quick closing date and secured it as an investment project.

I called the daughter, Tahlia, and she was happy to take it even if it meant some painting being done around her. We helped her move in and get settled. I realised she and I had a lot in common as we got to know each other better during workout sessions. Like me, she had an interest in Buddhism, loved to keep fit and enjoyed cooking healthy food. We became firm friends.

Trev began working long hours at the new rental property in order to complete the reno. I helped out when I could, but my numerous commitments meant I was not there much. And so, despite our best efforts, the two weeks of planned renovation work stretched out to more than six weeks. Tahlia didn't seem to mind. If anything, she seemed more than happy Trev was putting in extra hours to make the house look like it should feature in the next issue of *Homes & Gardens*.

In the middle of all this, I received a call from the chronic cerebrospinal venous insufficiency research team in Melbourne informing me that my third trial surgical procedure had been booked for the following month. The procedure was fairly routine now. They would insert a wire and a balloon into the jugular vein in my neck in order to widen it. As good old fate would have it, the surgery was scheduled smack dab on my 40th birthday. I wondered if I should ask them to change the date based on my previous history, then told myself, *Nah, Kat, stop being a paranoid drama queen, everything will be fine.* In hindsight, I should have trusted my intuition.

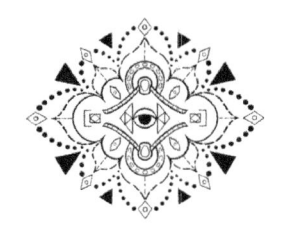

CHAPTER THIRTY-FIVE
Liberation Therapy

Focus on your strengths, not your weaknesses.
Focus on your character, not your reputation.
Focus on your blessings, not your misfortunes.
~ Roy T. Bennett

Just like my marriage to Trevor, CCSVI began as a love story and ended up mired in controversy and chaos. It was 1995, and Elena Ravalli was living a charmed life in the historic Italian city of Ferrara. In recent months, however, the seemingly healthy 37-year-old had experienced a series of strange attacks of vertigo, numbness, temporary vision loss, and crushing fatigue. She saw her doctor, who referred her to the local hospital for more tests. Elena was diagnosed with multiple sclerosis. Her husband, Paolo Zamboni, was devastated. But unlike most people, Zamboni had an ace up his sleeve.

During the 15th and 16th centuries, Ferrara had been an intellectual and artistic centre of excellence, attracting the greatest minds of the Italian Renaissance. The tradition continued in the form of the University of Ferrara, where Zamboni held the post of Professor of Medicine. He vowed to solve the mystery of MS and cure his wife of the disease. He scoured dusty books, researched centuries-old sources and consulted with his peers, eventually putting forward a radical idea. Zamboni suggested compromised blood flow in the veins draining the central nervous system was causing a build-up of iron in the brain, triggering an autoimmune reaction.

He did an ultrasound of his wife's neck, along with some other MS patients, and made a startling discovery: They all had partially blocked or occluded veins. He immediately scheduled his wife for a venoplasty operation. It worked! Her symptoms eased, many even disappeared, and she stopped having further attacks. And so, the theory of chronic cerebrospinal venous insufficiency was born. Zamboni later called it his 'liberation therapy'. It made headlines around the world as a miracle cure for MS.

Fast forward to Australia a decade or so later. On my quest to find a cure for MS, I stumbled across Professor Thompson, who was performing CCSVI procedures in Melbourne. After having an ultrasound done on my neck he informed me I did indeed have partially blocked veins and booked me for the procedure the following week.

But the night before the surgery was due, Professor Thompson called me personally, saying the hospital board had banned him from doing any further procedures on MS patients until a proper trial was completed and that my surgery had been indefinitely postponed. Frustrated and disappointed, I drove back to Jrudgerie and went down the path of stem cell therapy instead.

I consigned CCSVI to the dustbin of history, along with snake venom, hyperbaric oxygen chambers, anticoagulants, and histamine desensitisation therapy. Out of the blue, five years later, I received a call from the professor's research team at the Alfred Hospital in Melbourne. They had finally received the green light to conduct a CCSVI trial for MS patients. It would consist of four procedures six months apart. Would I be interested in being a part of it?

By now I'd undergone stem cell therapy and been relapse-free for five years. Even so, my brain and spinal cord were scarred from previous attacks and I was far from 'normal' in terms of my physical capabilities. I jumped at the chance to be part of the trial, knowing the issue of partially blocked veins in my neck could cause a relapse. Controversy was swirling in the media about whether CCSVI actually helped MS patients or not, as a number of new trials showed conflicting results. Dr Zamboni was being called a fraud in some quarters. I decided it was still worth a shot.

Once again I drove to Melbourne to await my fate. No late-night, last-minute call this time. The surgery went ahead as planned, but with one small caveat: it was a double-blind placebo trial. Neither the researchers nor I knew whether I was a placebo patient or a recipient of the real deal. The good news was, all the patients in the trial would eventually receive the venoplasty by the end of the second year.

At this stage in my life, I felt as if Zamboni's liberation therapy was being paralleled by a second liberation happening within my mind. A ten-year journey into Buddhism, yoga and meditation had finally rid my head of many of its neuroses. I was still a long way from attaining enlightenment, but at least I was no longer asleep at the wheel on the Highway to Suffering. Buddhists believe the path to liberation is a spiritual quest to find true happiness. I thought that was the coolest idea; that the meaning of life was simply to be happy and knowing that the only way to get there was to build a happiness bus and take everyone else along for the ride.

There was a tap on the front door, then I heard it open.

'Hey, it's me. I've got the dog and the vino!' Tahlia called out.

'Great, I'm in the kitchen. Hope you're hungry.'

The dog announced his arrival with loud barking. Almost immediately the kids ran excitedly out of their rooms to greet him.

'Barky!' they shouted in unison.

'Thanks so much guys for looking after Barky again. I'll only be gone a few days, and I'll give you scallywags some pocket money for walking him,' Tahlia offered gratefully.

The kids had always wanted a dog, but we travelled too much and I was not a dog person. Tahlia asked if she could occasionally leave the dog with me and Trev when she worked away, and we decided it was a good compromise. I was not a fan of Barky—he was barky by name and barky by nature—but the kids loved the mutt and the few extra dollars they earned for walking it, and Trevor seemed to enjoy having the dog around.

'How's the reno shaping up for you? Hopefully, it hasn't been too much of an inconvenience,' I said apologetically.

'It's going great, the place is looking spectacular! You are so lucky to have such a talented husband. Today he painted a coffee table for me that he said he made in high school. It's in my favourite shade of blue. Gosh, I wish I could find a guy like him.'

We watched through the kitchen window as the kids chased the dog around the trampoline.

With an air of wistfulness, Tahlia said, 'Your kids are so sweet!'

'Yes, most of the time they are, except when they're not.'

We both laughed. I asked, 'So tell me girl, have you met anyone interesting yet?'

It was a loaded question as I knew there were only about 2.5 single men in town. I didn't like her chances.

'Uh...no, not yet.'

'Well, good news! The horse races are next month. Single men will be coming in from everywhere, so I'm sure you'll meet a nice guy there.'

I cleaned two wine glasses with a tea towel, filled them with a generous serving of savage plonk, aka sauvignon blanc, and passed one to Tahlia. I hung the tea towel back up and smiled at the embroidered reminder to *Never Let A Good Disaster Go To Waste*. I raised my glass.

'To finding you a hot guy,' I said and clinked her glass against mine as we locked eyes.

'To finding the right guy,' she murmured back, looking past me at the kids playing in the backyard.

Just then we heard Trev's car pull up. Barky and the kids raced out to greet him. After navigating the chaos, he strolled into the kitchen, gave me a peck on the cheek and set down his paint-splattered lunch box next to the sink.

'Hey Tahl,' he acknowledged casually as he grabbed a cold beer from the fridge. 'I finished off that table for you. I think you're gonna love it.'

I felt a pang of irritation rise up. Last week it was a cosy breakfast nook, this week the coffee table. The project was starting to blow out timewise. I forced myself to quell my rising anger. After all, he was doing an amazing job and had been putting in some really long hours at the house trying to get the project completed.

'I'm painting the roof tomorrow,' he announced.

'What colour?' I asked, then bit my tongue.

The outside colours of the house had been the source of many a disagreement as of late. Although Tahlia was diplomatically keeping out of it, she secretly admitted to agreeing with my colour choices.

Trev looked at me defiantly.

'Mission Brown.'

'Seriously? Mission Brown?'

It took all my 'disappearing irritating person' effort to not beat him with a tea towel and have the conversation dissolve into an argument.

Tahlia looked at both of us and decided it was time to go.

'I'll leave you two to it. Good luck with Barky.'

I asked, 'Aren't you staying for dinner?'

'Better not, I've got a big day tomorrow.'

Trev walked her out. He returned, grabbed another cold beer and silently retreated to the back veranda. I was left with shouting kids, a barking dog and vegetables that needed peeling. I sighed. *Joyful effort, Kitty, joyful effort!*

The annual horse races were a huge social event for Jrudgerie. People drove in from everywhere, literally quadrupling the town's population overnight. Trev had, in his wisdom, decided to celebrate my 40th birthday early by having a party for me at the races. To be honest, I didn't enjoy big celebrations in my honour, even if a horse race broke out in the middle of it. I would have rather gone on a yoga retreat, but for Trev my 40th was an excuse for an epic weekend on the piss.

All up, around 80 people came to the celebration in the marquee we'd hired on the rails of the track. A decadent chocolate birthday cake was served, which made up for the fact that I was avoiding overindulging in the champagne. Despite my initial reservations, I really enjoyed the day, partly because I could remember it for once as I wasn't drinking and partly because, well, country races are fun and this was the most exciting annual event to occur in Jrudgerie.

When the races finally wound down around 5 p.m., Trev invited everyone back to our house for a bonfire. By this stage he was well on his way to being smashed, and all I wanted was to go home and chill out. But there was nothing I could do about it so I reluctantly joined in with the bonfire party and played hostess. At some stage Tahlia showed up, just as I was sneaking away to curl up and watch a movie in bed.

'Hey, sorry I'm so late,' Tahlia apologised. 'Work—you know how it is.'

'No worries. Feel free to go out back and join in with the party. I'm heading to Melbourne tomorrow to be ready for my surgery bright and early Monday morning.'

Two days later I pulled into the car park of the Alfred Hospital in Melbourne. The sun was just peeking above the buildings of the city. It was a typical crisp, spring day. 'Happy birthday,' I whispered to myself as I walked up to the admission counter. The first thing I noticed was its colour: Mission Brown. There goes the universe taunting me again I noted, amused.

After I signed all the paperwork and was being prepped for surgery, an orderly parked me outside the swinging doors of Operating Theatre 3. I was lying on a gurney wearing nothing but a flimsy hospital gown, feeling incredibly grateful. Once again I was being given the opportunity to be a pioneer for ground-breaking MS therapy. I was a warrior, not a victim.

I began wondering how the next chapter of my life would play out. I was pretty sure I'd been a placebo up until now and marvelled at the power of the placebo effect. Such a perfect example of the power of the mind and how your perception paints your reality. I thought about my marriage and family. Trev had been so sweet to organise a birthday bash for me, even though I would've been content with an 'updo' and a black-and-white polka dot dress from an op shop.

Our lives were getting easier, even though we'd had some big fights and tough times. It wasn't really any different from what most couples went through, but now that the kids were getting older it wouldn't be long before we could finally fulfil our dream of living on the coast. I'd finally claim back my surfer dude! He still had a fit, strong body even though the golden locks were long gone—he was now as bald as a badger. Hell, I might even be able to run down the beach again with my kids if the CCSVI therapy was successful.

In summary, I was trying to give the concept of happiness and joy in my life a red-hot go. I knew it still required lots of practice, discipline and patience and that I probably had to settle for lesser versions of happiness first, but I was determined to make it happen. Buddhism defines the first level of happiness as *santosha*, contentment; the second level as *sukha*, a deep-seated sense of well-being; the third level as *mudita*, joy, an irrepressible elation about life; and the fourth level as *ananda*, bliss, ecstasy. Without the assistance of chocolate and champagne, I was probably sitting somewhere near *santosha*, with the occasional foray into *sukha* and *mudita*. And I was okay with that.

My daydream was interrupted by the operating room door swinging open and a nurse telling me they'd be ready for me in ten minutes. I smiled. This was it, the start of my new life. My liberation.

Moments later my mobile vibrated against my leg. I looked at the screen. It was my home number.

'Morning, Mummy,' Stella said happily. My heart warmed. She proceeded to sing me 'Happy Birthday', then excitedly announced, 'And guess what mummy?'

'Yes darling?'

'Tahlia slept over in your bed last night!'

My birthday disaster had begun.

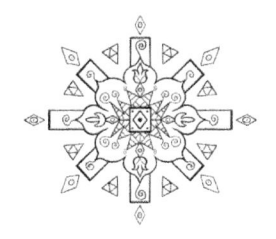

CHAPTER THIRTY-SIX
Life After Life

'I am a lover of what is, not because I'm a spiritual person, but because it hurts when I argue with reality.'
~ Byron Katie

Living in the fishbowl of a small town in rural New South Wales is tricky enough when everything is going right, but when your life is turned upside down by a major betrayal the fishbowl becomes a magnifying glass.

This was my predicament in the days and weeks following my marriage breakdown. After all, it wasn't as though Trevor and his new girlfriend Tahlia could avoid me. There were three kids involved, the town only had one main street and a total of 800 residents, and Tahlia was living just up the road from me in a rental house I half-owned and had helped renovate. Hell, I'd even chosen the rug on her bedroom floor.

For the residents of Jrudgerie, Trev's affair was the scandal of the year: the beloved son of a well-known local farming family dumping the outsider Canadian who the entire community had rallied around to save from a life of disease and disability. The news spread like wildfire. I tried to hold my head high and carry on with my life as usual, but it was impossible to ignore the curious stares. Some people offered me their condolences and sympathy while others avoided me or the topic altogether.

To say being the subject of a sex scandal was humiliating would be an understatement. People treated me as if someone I loved had been murdered, and in a way they were right. My previous identity had been ripped away and buried, replaced by another. I was no longer 'the wife', I was the 'estranged partner'. We were a broken family in a town uncharacteristically full of happy, whole ones.

It took all my might to keep my thoughts focused on gratitude, to recognise what was actually going right for me each day, even if sometimes all I could find were small things, like a hot shower or my car starting. As for Tahlia, I'm sure many people in my position would have revelled in painting her as a homewrecker, but I wasn't one of them. To err is human, to forgive radically is divine. I wished her no ill will.

Why? Because I recognised that harbouring hate in my heart would have only created bad karma for myself. I'd also had plenty of time to analyse the betrayal and acknowledge my role in the ending of the marriage. It wasn't easy to admit, but I was often angry and short-tempered. I hadn't put enough effort and time into keeping the spark alive, resulting in us slowly drifting apart. I'd focused more on my work and children than my husband. I preferred to do a hundred sweaty sit-ups at the gym over a romantic dinner out.

Clearly, that didn't give Trevor the right to do what he did, but by taking ownership of my situation, by not adopting a victim mentality or a blame-game mindset, I could respond rather than react to my husband's brutal betrayal. I needed to take positive steps to ensure a better future not just for myself but for all of us. This was important to me. My children would have to deal with the fallout from this break-up just as much as I would. I likened it to the doughnut lesson I'd learnt as a kid. Being unhappy about someone else's happiness wasn't going to help me be a happy person. Conversely, being happy about someone's unhappiness would never bring more happiness into my life.

I worked hard every day to follow through with my positive mindset. I told myself the end of my marriage and split-up of my family didn't need to be thought of as a tragedy. Rather, it could be considered a form of liberation therapy, an opening up of new opportunities and possibilities, another chance to learn about impermanence and cultivate empathy for all those going through something similar.

Of course, there were times when I fell off the wagon and made disparaging remarks about Trev to friends. There were also days when loneliness overwhelmed me. Getting over betrayal in 12 hours didn't mean my life was all unicorns and daisies. It still sucked sometimes, but I actively tried to choose a better path and stick to the 12 principles, which meant being mindful of my words and actions and consciously remembering to send good thoughts Trevor and Tahlia's way every time I wanted to do the exact opposite.

Thankfully they reacted in kind, and together we worked diligently to make the best of an awkward situation. Trev avoided stoking the flames of the gossip bonfire by moving to his parent's farm, and the kids seamlessly bounced between the farm and my house each week without restriction. I did my yoga and nutrition classes as if nothing had happened and even let Trev continue to conduct his boxing classes from the home gym. It all just fell into place.

I couldn't help but marvel at how well we were getting along. Okay, so we weren't singing 'Kumbaya' together, but there was a certain level of understanding and respect. I was loving my newfound freedom, along with the extra closet space and the fact I had a lot less laundry to do. The steps I'd applied to overcome my betrayal in 12 hours provided me with benefits far beyond just peace of mind. Friends commented about how well I was taking it all, how great I looked. I was praised for taking the high road, I was told how wonderful it was that I'd chosen to be accepting and gracious rather than bitter and distraught. I had a real sense of pride at how well I was handling life. The lack of tension, anger and resentment between me, Trevor and Tahlia made it easy for the kids to navigate the changing circumstances of our home life. We were winning at the separation game. Until it all came crashing down on top of me like a ton of karmic bricks a few short weeks later.

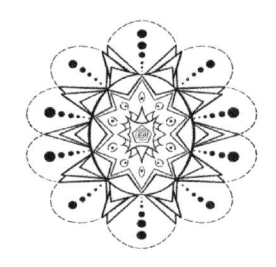

CHAPTER THIRTY-SEVEN
Releasing the Karma Genie

The tongue has no bones but is strong enough to break a heart.
So be careful with your words.
~ Ashu

With the separation moving along so amicably, I convinced myself that we had all transitioned seamlessly to something approaching mutual acceptance. As such, I fell into a sense of complacency. Many of the items on my to-do list following our split slowly began slipping away into the background. One of these was the changing of my personal banking passwords.

When I finally tackled the issue I was in for one hell of a shock. I should've known that life doesn't travel in a linear progression. What was it Lama Marut said? *You're either in a disaster or between them.* In my case, I found out Trevor had withdrawn $30,000 from our joint mortgage account without my knowledge or consent. I was stunned. This *had* to be a mistake. Confused, I checked the statement again, but there they were: six withdrawals of $5,000 each over the course of the last three weeks, the first dating back to my 40th birthday.

It was a big chunk of the money my Czech Nana had given me for my inheritance. Hell had nothing on my fury.

I lost it large. It was late on a Monday afternoon when I discovered the missing money. Trevor was due to teach a boxing class from the studio at our house, and as fate would have it, he pulled up outside my door moments later. I charged into the street.

'You lying, cheating, fucking thief!' I screamed, kicking his idling ute.

Trevor was stunned, unsure what was happening. All he knew was that his wife, who up to now had handled their break-up rather gracefully, had temporarily gone insane.

'You stole money from our mortgage account, you bastard.'

The lightbulb suddenly went on.

'Calm down, I can explain,' he pleaded.

'Really? How exactly do you explain using my passwords to take out thirty grand from our account? That was an inheritance from my grandmother, you fucker.'

Trev clearly didn't fancy being called a fucker in public. His face turned red and his eyes narrowed.

'I was owed that money,' he spat. 'Look at all the work I've done on the rental property, and…and…what about all the renovations I've done on our house, the one you're living in now?'

'Are you joking me? You want me to pay you for doing household chores and repairs around the family house?' I asked, incredulous. 'What about the thousands of hours of unpaid work I've done over the years?'

I knew this argument would end up in Nowheresville. He had his story and was sticking to it—the hard-done-by husband who'd worked long hours without pay—and I had mine—the faithful wife who'd sacrificed everything to stay and raise a family in Jrudgerie. It had been the basis for many arguments prior to the affair. It always ended in a stalemate.

'Guess what, sweetheart,' he sneered. 'I don't need to put up with your bullshit anymore.'

He glared at me as he took off, tires squealing. A few people who'd shown up for Trev's boxing class were staring at me with a mixture of shock and excitement. They hadn't realised their class would include ringside seats to 'fight night on the footpath'.

Following Trev's sudden departure everyone retreated to their cars and drove off, leaving me standing in the street with my hands tightly gripping my hair. Fuuuck! I turned to go inside. It was only then I noticed my daughter Stella at the living room window, tears streaking her sweet, innocent face. Oh my God, what have I done?

The shame of acting like a lunatic in front of my daughter and the neighbourhood made me rein in my anger, at least temporarily. With a huge effort I gained control of myself and cooked dinner for Stella and my new boarder, Kathryn. Deep down there was still a seething, burning rage churning inside me. That night I did the worst thing possible for my future happiness. I left Stella at home with Kathryn and went to the pub, drank too much and proceeded, in my inebriated state, to tell anyone who would listen that my husband was not only a liar and a cheat but also a thief.

My words and actions were in complete contradiction to everything I'd been striving for. In the space of one night I ruined all the good work I'd done to overcome the initial betrayal and keep things amicable between Trev and I. I justified this by telling myself that although I could rationalise his cheating, I couldn't rationalise his theft of the money. For me it represented a whole new level of betrayal and caused my anger to erupt like Krakatoa. What was it Saint Augustine said? Resentment is like drinking poison and waiting for the other person to die. My husband wouldn't have been so eloquent. He would have simply said, 'I guess karma really is a bitch.'

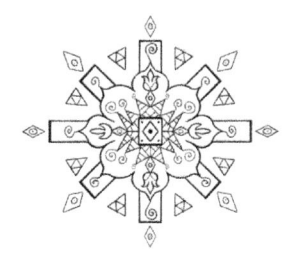

CHAPTER THIRTY-EIGHT
The Five Rs

We are not privy to the stories behind people's actions, so we should be patient with others and suspend judgement of them, recognising the limits of our understanding.
- Epictetus

The repercussions of my fall from grace, in particular my drunken night at the pub telling all and sundry that my husband was a liar, a cheat and a thief would come back to haunt me with a vengeance in the following days and weeks. I'd pulled the cork out of the bottle and let the karma genie free, and there was no putting it back in. I had poisoned the well, tarnished Trev's good name and reputation, and soon I would have to reap what I had sown. It was that simple.

As I lay in bed that night disillusioned, upset and sleepless, I meditated on dispelling my anger, the most toxic of all emotions. Buddha once said, 'Hatred can never be ceased by hatred, it can only be ceased by love. This is an eternal law.' I made a conscious decision to conquer my anger, my real enemy, before it consumed me. It was time to end the rage in the cage and get angry with my anger. I reminded myself I couldn't change what I'd said and done in the pub. That toothpaste was never going back in the tube. But what I could do was admit my mistake and make amends. I remembered the Five Rs Maree told me about and that Buddhists use to dispel anger and avoid the cycle of suffering: Recognise, Regret, Recompense, Rejoice and Remember.

I knew Trev wouldn't have taken the money if he didn't believe he was entitled to it, even if I thought his reasons were asinine. More importantly, I needed to learn the lesson from my disastrous outburst and do my best not to disparage anyone in the future.

I carefully examined why I was so frustrated and angry. Of course, I was pissed that I'd just been taken for a huge sum of money, but I was also angry at myself for inadvertently allowing this to happen. My grandfather, Papa Joe, always said, 'Never put off until tomorrow what you can do today.' And what had I done? The complete opposite. I'd put off changing my passwords countless times over the last few weeks. Could have, should have, would have, but didn't—that was the reality. And there was no arguing with reality, or karma. I was now reaping what I had sown. Cause and effect, action and reaction. I called the bank the next day. They explained there was nothing they could do about the withdrawals. I'd committed a mortal banking sin by sharing my personal password with my partner. I'd essentially given Trev permission to take out the money.

My mobile rang a few minutes later. It was Trev's mum. She was upset.

'I've heard you've been saying things about my son around town. You have no idea how much this has hurt me and my family.'

Then she hung up. I was stunned. She had never spoken to me so angrily! A few hours later I received a text from Trev informing me he would no longer pay his share of the kids' yearly boarding and school fees. It also became clear in the following days his father would not talk to me anymore, and I stopped receiving invites to family gatherings. It was immediate and harsh payback. I remembered one of my favourite sayings when I was a teenager waking up hungover after a big night out: 'Last night at midnight I felt immense, but now I feel like twenty cents.'

I nearly cried in frustration. All I could do about Trev's parents was continue practising the Five Rs and apologise for my actions. The kids' schooling was another issue entirely.

Both older boys, Luke and Jack, were happily attending a Catholic boarding school. The local high school was not a good fit for them for various reasons, but I also wanted them to have a foundation of Christian values, a moral compass to guide them through their teenage years. I felt strongly about this because when I was their age I'd squandered my chance to follow through with schooling. My father always placed great importance on education and had done his best to keep me in line, but even so I barely made it through high school and never pursued university. I felt I was better off working and having money than being a poor student. I didn't want that to happen to my kids, not that I had any regrets. I believed they deserved to have the option of choosing to go to university or not, and private school was one giant leap towards that goal.

Trev, on the other hand, made it clear he was against the idea of sending the boys to boarding school. He wanted the kids at home and felt it was a waste of money.

'The local school was good 'nuf for me, and it'll be good 'nuf for me kids,' he'd repeatedly argue.

'Case in point,' I'd say. 'You can't even speak proper English.' As a boxer, perhaps Trev had been hit in the head too many times to believe an education was important. He figured that withdrawing his financial support would make it impossible for me to pay the private school fees on my own. He was so confident about winning the fight, he told me he was enrolling both boys in the local high school for the following year. But he seriously underestimated my willpower and determination.

CHAPTER THIRTY-NINE
Love Is a Verb as Well as a Noun

Throw me to the wolves and I will come back leading the pack.
~ Katness, The Hunger Games (quoting Seneca)

In the wake of our nasty fallout, I could've easily hitched my wagon to the 'poor me, single mother' paradigm following Trev's decision to withdraw his financial support for the boys' private school fees. I could've become angry with him all over again, blamed the world for the fact I didn't have enough money, caved to his demands, and sent my boys to the local high school. But I refused to give up or adopt a victim mentality.

Rather, I decided to actively embrace the challenge of becoming a 'successful single mother'. I ramped up my yoga, fitness, Pilates, and nutrition programs. I took in boarders. I used my extensive sales training and passion for healthy eating to sell Thermomixes—high-tech German cooking machines. I read self-help books and listened to motivational podcasts. I whispered Tony Robbins quotes to myself before going to sleep at night. And I discovered that being in a small rural town wasn't a curse at all but a blessing.

No one else was doing what I was doing, either in Jrudgerie or the surrounding area. I had no competition, people knew and respected me, they recommended me to friends and family. Best of all, it was cheap to live in Jrudgerie and the lack of shops and entertainment meant I could devote all my spare time to work rather than to socialising and shopping.

When I combined this with a lifetime of frugal spending habits, mostly instilled in me by my parents but also by my extensive Buddhist training, I soon earned enough to not only pay all the school fees for my boys but be financially independent as well. I was incredibly proud of myself. I'd achieved what I set out to do and, more importantly, set an example for my children. Barriers only exist if you choose to believe they do.

One of the many beautiful concepts Buddhism teaches you about money is that the desire to be self-sufficient and provide for your family is not inherently selfish, especially if it puts you in a better position to help others in a positive way. However, having a scarcity mindset, constantly comparing yourself to others and living in fear of not having enough stops you from creating a life of abundance, contentment and happiness. The trick is to say to yourself, 'If I really want it, I will find a way, but do I really need it?' Lama Marut had a perfect mantra around this concept that was as simple as it was profound: 'Om, I have enough, ah hum.' Meaning exactly that. I have enough money. I have enough clothes. I have enough cars. I have enough room in my home. I have enough friends. I have enough job success. I have enough entertainment. I have enough of everything to be happy. Full stop!

I recalled one day driving an 800 km round trip to do a cooking demonstration for Thermomix. All told, the endeavour took more than 12 hours and I never sold a single machine. But because I was not attached to the outcome or the money, I still walked away happy. I knew that if I viewed it as doing a service for others, if I carried it out with joyful effort, I would be content no matter what.

Two of the biggest lessons I learned going through my divorce was that wealth does not always guarantee you happiness and expecting everything to go your way will cause you suffering if you attach too strongly to the outcomes. Sometimes you can win the battle but still lose the war. There's always a price to pay.

Although I was intent on trying to recoup the $30,000 Trev had 'taken' from me, I decided to steer clear of the courts and lawyers. I also decided not to allow myself to become overly stressed or attached to the outcomes of the divorce. I applied an attitude of joyful effort to the whole situation.

Trev proposed a settlement, which I agreed to, and the boys remained at their school, but I never did get back my $30,000. The good news was, I saved twice that sum by staying away from the family law courts. I also realised something life-changing in the process. Love is a verb as well as a noun. You can choose to love as well as send love. Equally, you can choose to hate as well as send hate. Hating and loving take equal amounts of energy but carry significantly different outcomes. In my case, choosing to send love to Trev and Tahlia allowed me to reach a point where my happiness and contentment was not contingent on the actions of others. And my choice to go with love eventually rewarded me with a trip to the city of love—Paris!

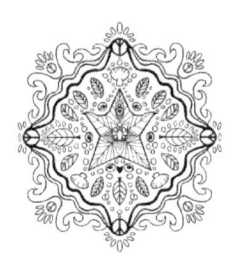

CHAPTER FORTY
A Backpack Full of Bowling Balls

*Let us rise up and be thankful, for if we didn't learn a lot at least we
learned a little, and if we didn't learn a little, at least we didn't get sick,
and if we got sick, at least we didn't die; so, let us all be thankful.*
- Buddha

I arrived in Europe on my 41st birthday with a very excited 11-year-old Stella in tow. She was going to hang out with my childhood friend Sandra, who I'd worked with in Italy, while I attended the four-day Thermomix event in Paris. Afterwards, Stella and I would travel together to the south of Spain and wander from village to village, learning Spanish, eating tapas and indulging in sangria—or at least I would anyway!

I'd come a long way since my previous birthday when I'd been grappling with the fallout of a philandering husband, a friend who'd deceived me and fears of being a broke, single mother. By choosing to take responsibility for my future in those initial 12 hours after the betrayal and sticking to my 12 principles in the days and months that followed, I managed to completely turn that vision around.

I embraced the world of Thermomix and cooked my way to the top of the sales ladder using every tool at my disposal: my coupon cult sales experience, my extensive knowledge of nutrition and my philosophy of cooking simple, wholesome food quickly and with a minimum of fuss. The fact I'd owned a Thermomix for years and understood implicitly that they weren't just pricey German blenders but gateways to a universe of healthy cooking also helped immensely! And the reward for all my hard-earned efforts? A luxury, all-expenses-paid trip to France, along with 50 other top consultants from around Australia. God with an R would have been proud! It seemed the first step of my thousand-mile journey to overcome my betrayal had actually led me a thousand miles away to a place where I could savour the sweetness of my success.

And France was sweet indeed, home to buttery croissants, a seemingly infinite variety of cheeses and wines, decadent chocolates, and, most important of all, Vorwerk's Thermomix factory. Located 150 km southwest of Paris next to the famous 15th-century chateau, Montigny-le-Gannelon, it was the epitome of German efficiency. After enjoying a highly anticipated tour of the factory, we were ushered into a world of food-laden, hedonistic indulgence.

We dined at Michelin-starred restaurants, had private food and wine tours of ancient chateaus, gorged on macaroons and petit fours at Versailles, enjoyed a dinner cruise on the Seine, and took in a private fashion show with hors d'oeuvres at the beautiful Galeries Lafayette on the Champs-Élysées. By the time all the shows and gastronomic over-indulgences were finished, I was three kilos heavier and ready to do some exercise in Spain.

I picked up Stella from Sandra's place, and we winged it to Madrid. A few days of sightseeing, complete with plenty of sangria and sides of the local dish, *patatas bravas*, eventually led us to a train that whisked us away to the gorgeous seaside town of Cadiz. Stella and I marvelled at the architecture and the cobblestone roads. According to our guide book, the roads were constructed by the Romans more than 2,000 years earlier. We were hoping the current road we were strolling along would lead us to the AirBnB we'd booked into for the night.

There was just one small problem. I'd become overwhelmed with an acute case of vertigo and could barely walk. My backpack felt like it was full of bowling balls that had somehow come alive and decided to have a party. Also, I couldn't seem to focus my eyes. The world around me had turned into a swirling blur. In a bid to correct my obscured vision I tried closing first one eye and then the other. It didn't work. I stumbled over a cobblestone and fell face-first onto the path, my hands and legs askew.

'Mum! What's wrong?' Stella cried, kneeling next to me.

The truth was, I had no idea. I'd never experienced anything like this before.

'Mum, are you okay?' Stella pleaded for an answer. I lay still a moment, hoping a troupe of handsome Spanish matadors would magically appear to help me out of my predicament. But when they didn't materialise I summoned up my remaining energy and hauled myself to my feet.

'I'm okay, but I think I'm going to need your help.'

Stella removed my backpack and heaved it onto her chest. She already had her own bag on her back. She looked like a turtle sandwiched between two shells. Although she was tiny, she was tuff. If only I still had my favourite childhood t-shirt to give her. I did my best to stagger alongside her without falling over again. Poor Stell, in her short life she'd lifted me off the ground more times than I could count. Once—twice, tops—it was due to an overindulgence of champagne, but usually it was because of my issues with MS.

I had no intention of wasting our holiday checking into a hospital for what would no doubt be a series of exhaustive tests, so I decided to find a happy place for us to hole up until our flight back to Australia the following week. I Googled yoga and horse riding, our two favourite passions, and to my delight up popped a health retreat featuring both and located in the mountains near Cadiz. Perfect!

Over the next week Stella and I glamped in a luxury tent at the health retreat. I did yoga as best I could and chilled out the rest of the time while Stella rode horses and hung out in the stables. In between we dined on delicious raw, healthy food. At the end of the week I felt rejuvenated and even worked out how to walk in a straight line by keeping one eye partially closed. Unfortunately, the dizziness continued unabated, so I didn't push it by indulging in sangria.

When Stell and I returned from Spain, I went straight in to see my GP, and he gave me some drugs to counteract the dizziness. I was hoping I had Ménière's disease or some other form of inner ear problem or maybe even a viral infection. But none of the drugs worked, and a viral infection was ruled out.

'You know, there's only a couple of other options to explain this, Kat,' my GP stated, using the soft, neutral tones of a doctor about to deliver bad news.

I stared at him intently, my mind spinning with thoughts and emotions. I was hoping he was going to say brain tumour, syphilis or cancer. Anything would've been more welcome than the alternative I could see was coming.

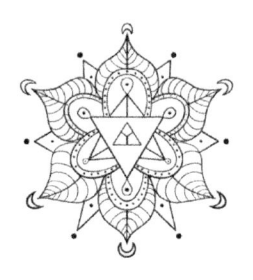

CHAPTER FORTY-ONE
Struggling With My Big Girl Pants

When facing adversity, we may think we've reached our limit, but actually the more trying the circumstances, the closer we are to making a breakthrough. The darker the night, the nearer the dawn. Victory in life is decided by that last concentrated burst of energy filled with the resolve to win.
~ Daisaku Ikeda

There's a wise Buddhist proverb that says in order to progress along the path to happiness and contentment, you need to fully accept the present. Funny how it sounds so easy in theory but when faced with a potentially life-changing moment, especially one involving a serious health issue, it becomes exponentially harder to accept. Screw it, I thought, let's get this over with. I gave my GP an imperceptible nod to continue. There was no dodging this bullet.

'Kat, taking into account the dizziness, the blurred vision, the lack of motor control in your limbs, and your medical history, everything points to a relapse. I'm so sorry to have to tell you this, but...your MS has come back.'

And there it was. My imagined fears had now coalesced into hard fact. There were only a few things in life I prayed would never return: neon clothing, acid-wash jeans and MS. I had been disease-free for six glorious years, but it seemed any protection I'd been afforded by the MSCs had now faded away.

A few hours later I was lying in a bed in Jrudgerie's hospital, better known locally as God's Waiting Room, watching my doctor insert a cannula into my arm.

'Nice veins,' the doctor commented. 'We don't get many young, plump ones like that around here.'

'Oh, um, thanks,' I stammered, not sure whether to take it as a compliment. The cannula was attached via a clear tube to an IV bag full of methylprednisolone, a powerful steroid I'd taken countless times before to counteract my MS attacks. I willed the steroids to do their job and put an end to the dizziness so I could check the hell out before the kitchen began serving the next meal of puréed meat and potatoes. But just in case the drugs didn't work, in the corner was a wheelchair.

This was my worst nightmare, a situation I swore I'd never let myself reach. Yet here I was, in my 40s, divorced, alone, lying in a bed in a de facto nursing home with no husband to hold my hand because he was now holding Tahlia's, and with a wheelchair prepped for me. It took every ounce of effort to fight back the tears of disappointment, frustration and anger welling up inside, threatening to burst out. Worst of all was the feeling of having failed. I'd let down my children, my family, my friends, all the people who'd donated time and money to help me with my quest to find a cure. I'd gambled everything on this radical alternative therapy, and now it appeared I had to start all over again.

I thought back to something Maree, my Buddhist mentor, once told me when I was struggling with my meditation practice:

'You may think this is boring and a waste of time, but we meditate to train our brains, to become an observer of our thoughts and to master our minds. This in turn helps us recognise the challenges confronting us every day and deal with them in a positive, proactive manner. By choosing what thoughts to believe, we can tell ourselves a new and better story.'

Right now I was wallowing in self-pity and doubt. I was telling myself I was a failure rather than accepting the reality of my situation. Lama Marut's classically simple but powerful Buddhist mantra popped into my head: 'It's like this now.' Easy to say; not so easy to accept when the shit hits the fan. I sighed. I knew damn well what he'd say in response to this.

'It's just as important to do meditation and learn detachment and contentment in the good times as it is in the bad times. It's practice for showtime. And that's why you should never let a good disaster go to waste, because that's when the best lessons are learnt, that's when you need to pull on your big boy pants and put your spiritual muscles to the test.'

It was now showtime and I was struggling with my big boy pants—or in my case, my big girl pants. I forced myself to pause the negativity and reassess my situation in light of my Buddhist worldview. This was no time to feel sorry for myself. I had access to the best medical care, I had a good support network of friends, I was financially secure and I had kids and a family who loved me. What I needed to do now was find a way to 'cure' my disease all over again. I thought about my 'get out of jail free card', my booster vial full of purified MSCs sitting frozen in a lab overseas. Yes, all was not lost! It was time to play that card and buy my way back into the game of life.

I immediately called my former team of Israeli doctors, only to be informed the procedure was now considered obsolete and they could no longer use my frozen cells. Instead, they were harvesting MSCs from belly fat. Happy days I thought, take as many of them as you like. I'll even donate extra! But then the team hit me with the kicker. For various reasons, the cost of the procedure had gone up from $40,000 to $100,000.

Damn them to hell, I thought as I slammed down the phone. There goes my half-price deal. I was fuming. My MSCs had bought me over half a decade of perfect health and helped repair some of the destroyed bits of my brain and spinal cord. And now, just like that, they were gone.

What to do? I needed a Plan C. I'd already turned over every stone, or so I thought. I called a friend involved in medical research. She gave me the contact number for a researcher running stem cell trials for MS in Australia. His initial assessment of my situation was sobering.

'At your age and with your history it's unlikely we could accept you into our trial. You no longer meet the requirements, I'm so sorry.'

'Oh,' I said, feeling like a senior citizen. Surely this couldn't be it? I'd fought so hard and so long. The options facing me were now stark. Unbidden, a vision of the lady in the wheelchair at the bachelor auction sprang to mind. There was no way I was going down that road, *no way*. There *had* to be another path forward.

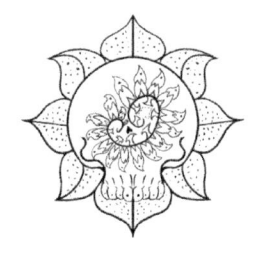

CHAPTER FORTY-TWO
Running Out of Kat Lives

*Do not judge me by my successes, judge me by how many times
I fell down and got back up again.*
~ Nelson Mandela

It's never easy when you throw your last roll of the dice and come up with a one-two combo rather than double sixes. Given the insanely high cost of pursuing alternative treatments overseas, my hope of yet another miraculous recovery from MS was fading fast. Then the MS researcher who I was still on the phone with and who had just informed me I was ineligible for the stem cell trials, threw me a lifeline.

'You know Kat, you may not be eligible for stem cell therapy, but there may be another option. It's called Lemtrada...'

Lemtrada? I hadn't heard about this drug.

'Alemtuzumab,' he clarified. 'A powerful drug, similar to chemo. It's been used since the early 2000s for chronic lymphocytic leukaemia, but just last month it was approved by the Pharmaceutical Benefits Scheme as a treatment for MS. It's heavy-duty and can have some nasty side effects, but none of them are as bad as having MS. If I were you, I'd give it a go. Clinical trials have been very promising. Some people have no new relapses, and the drug may also slow down the build-up of disability. Best of all, the costs are covered by the government.'

'Well,' I responded, relieved, 'that sounds perfect. Let's run with that.'

I dreaded returning to my neuro, the man who'd crushed my hopes so many years ago, but as they say...the devil you know. Interestingly, he'd had a change of perspective in the interim. My absence for more than six years due to good health had been duly noted, and he was now not nearly as sceptical about stem cells as he was before.

'I've had a relapse,' I admitted begrudgingly. 'A stem cell procedure is my preferred option, but I don't qualify for the trials here in Australia, and it costs too much to go overseas. However, after researching Lemtrada, I've decided it's my best option.'

'Lemtrada, ah yes. I've just begun treating some of my MS patients with it. You understand it's eight infusions given over two years with five years of mandatory monthly blood testing? And there's a long list of possible acute and chronic side effects, including thyroid issues, blood disorders, kidney disease and—'

'Please stop,' I pleaded. 'Look, I'm aware of the risks involved. I'm a high-stakes gambler, and I'm happy to go ahead with this. But please, don't tell me any more. I feel like I'm in an American drug commercial. I prefer blissful ignorance to unpleasant possibilities.'

He nodded and smiled. 'You got it. And good luck, Kat. You're a strong-willed woman. No doubt you'll come through this just fine.'

As chance would have it, a few days after my 42nd birthday I received the first of eight infusions over five days. The three additional doses were administered 12 months later. All up, it cost the government $150,000. I crossed my fingers and hoped it would be worth it.

It was. Within a few weeks of the first infusions I began feeling much stronger. My balance improved, and I could walk without constantly tripping over. It was a small miracle. Four blissful disease-free years went by with no repercussions from the toxic chemo cocktail I'd flushed through my veins. I was quietly confident I'd beaten the odds of developing any nasty side effects. After all, I'd been through so much, surely life would cut me a break, right?

It was during one of my mandated monthly blood tests shortly after that the lab flagged a problem with my thyroid. I was highly dubious of the results. Normally, low thyroid function results in excessive tiredness. But I felt normal. Was there anything else that could explain the results? I went to the doctor and he said the only other random factor that could affect the testing was an excess of cabbage. Yes, apparently cabbage had a chemical within it that could affect the thyroid. Then the penny dropped—I'd eaten a whole cabbage the day before my blood test! Why a whole cabbage, I hear you ask? Because it's a negative calorie food you can chew for a long time to trick the brain into thinking you've eaten a lot. Phew, that explained it!

But less than a month later my throat began to swell and I became extremely lethargic—so much so that I passed out in the bathroom of my house in Jrudgerie while giving myself a spray tan. Let me explain. Stella and I were planning to fly to Canada for the Christmas holidays and I was hoping to exude a healthy 'Aussie glow'. Luckily Stella and Luke were home at the time and heard the crash as I fell to the floor. When they saw me lying there unconscious, they assumed I'd somehow managed to gas myself with tanning fumes.

They did their best to try and revive me by shaking me and yelling at me, but it didn't do any good. I could hear them and feel them, but for some reason I couldn't speak. I felt as though I was dying. It was actually a very pleasant, peaceful feeling. Stella was crying. In her panic she couldn't remember our address to give to the emergency operator. It was enough for me to force myself from my lethargy and slur, 'Sstop worrying yuu guys... only the guud die young.'

'But Mum, you're not good and you're not young,' Luke said.

Luke, like me, loves to add levity to dark situations.

The ambulance ferried me to the local hospital. By the time I arrived I was drifting in and out of consciousness. The doctor slapped a bunch of resuscitation pads on my chest and legs and had the ambulance rush me to a marginally better-equipped hospital in the next town. Ten minutes into the journey, I was wide awake and chatting cheerfully with the ambos as if nothing had happened. They were astounded. I explained that other than a ruined spray tan, I was perfectly fine.

The ambos ignored my request to turn around and drop me home. At the hospital my blood tests came back showing my thyroid levels were off the charts. A classic side effect of taking Lemtrada. Okay, at least I only had to deal with one bad side effect, I told myself. I went home armed with thyroxine and a Skype appointment with an endocrinologist.

The thyroxine helped, slowly but surely. Over the next week I suffered from occasional blackouts, but nothing like my first one. The endocrinologist informed me I had Hashimoto's disease, better known as hypothyroidism. My body's immune system was working against me, attacking my thyroid.

'Unfortunately, the level of thyroid hormones in your body dropped so low you went into a type of coma called myxedema. It's very rare and can kill you if left untreated. In fact, it would have killed you if you hadn't gone to the hospital. Consider yourself very lucky.'

So I really *had* been at death's door. Nice to know that if a similar incident happened again, it was going to be a relaxing way to kick the bucket.

The endocrinologist summed up my situation: 'Kat, you will have to take this drug for the rest of your life. Your thyroid is no longer functioning.'

And just like that, another part of me was gone. I was starting to feel like the Black Knight in *Monty Python and the Holy*

Grail. Time to once again don my spiritual boxing gloves and punch my way out. I decided if it was at all possible, I'd still fly to Canada with Stella in a few days' time and spend Christmas in the bosom of my loving family. There's no place like home for dealing with an existential crisis. I consulted my endocrinologist, who gave me the okay.

'Take the thyroxine, Kat, and maybe cut back on the cabbage!'

As Stella and I were being driven to the airport by my brother-in-law in Melbourne, my phone rang. It was my neuro. I put him on speaker.

'Kat, good morning. Where are you?' he asked brusquely.

'I'm in Melbourne, about to fly to Canada.'

'Listen, I've just received your latest blood results.'

'Yes, I know my thyroid is stuffed. I've been working with the endo and he says—'

'That's not why I'm calling,' he interrupted. 'Your blood platelet count has dropped dramatically. It's 39.'

Silence. None of us had any idea what that meant.

'Kat, it should be over 150. You need to be checking into a hospital, not an airport.'

Ah-ha! That explained why I was covered in massive bruises! In my head I counted how many 'Kat' lives I had left. I figured I still had one or two up my sleeve.

'Surely this can wait until I get to Canada,' I implored. 'It's only a 28-hour journey, give or take.'

My brother-in-law and daughter looked at me with wide-eyed horror. They couldn't believe I was even considering getting on the plane. My neuro, perhaps not used to having his professional opinion opposed so belligerently, broke the tense silence by reaffirming the severity of the situation.

'Kat, as far as I'm concerned, this is critical...do not get on that plane!

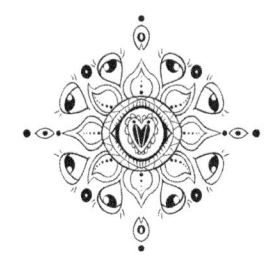

CHAPTER FORTY-THREE
The Domino Effect

Hardships often prepare ordinary people for an extraordinary destiny.
~ C.S. Lewis

My neurologist's announcement floored me for a few seconds. After being told by so many doctors that I was taking huge risks and should err on the side of safety, I tended to take their advice with a grain of salt. My strategy had worked so far—I was still alive after all.

I sat in the car on the outskirts of Tullamarine, Melbourne's international airport, mulling over my predicament. Dammit, what do I do now? I'd already pre-ordered my special in-flight meal. Okay, so it wasn't so much about the food or the money I'd lose as a result of a cancellation as much as it was about putting Stella in a compromising position on the flight if I fell deathly ill. Memories of my little girl picking me up off my knees in Cadiz sprang unbidden to mind. Stell was a lot bigger and stronger now. At the very least she could throw me onto a baggage trolley!

Stella was slowly shaking her head and looking at me disapprovingly. For the next few minutes we listened intently as the neuro explained my situation in greater detail.

'It sounds like you most likely have idiopathic thrombocytopenic purpura, or ITP, an auto-immune disorder that stops your blood from clotting. It's a well-known and potentially deadly side effect of Lemtrada.'

You have got to be frickin' kidding me, I muttered silently to myself.

'Okay, thanks for letting me know.'

I hung up, frustrated and annoyed but determined to find a second opinion. I called my GP in Jrudgerie. Living in a small outback town meant dealing with a revolving door of immigrant doctors who went to the country, where no one goes voluntarily, to expedite their immigration process. Our most recent doctor was Iraqi, a man I'd come to like and trust over the last few years. He was a good doctor, experienced, caring and not prone to overreaction. I trusted his advice. He took my call immediately.

I laid out my situation to him.

'The neuro has advised me not to go. What do you think? Can I make it?'

'Thirty-nine? That's pretty low, but you'll make it as long as you promise not to bump into anything or cut yourself badly along the way.'

'Sure, Doc, no problem.'

I smiled at my brother-in-law and Stella and gave them the thumbs-up. My brother-in-law shook his head, and Stella rolled her eyes in resignation. She knew better than to try to argue with me. I've always been the type of person who doesn't take no for an answer. It's what made me such a good salesperson.

Luckily for both of us, the journey was uneventful—well, if you don't count the one small episode where I briefly slipped into an unconscious state halfway across the Pacific. Stella stayed calm and kept an eye on me and didn't alert the stewardess. I recovered about ten minutes later, none the worse for my experience and no one the wiser around me.

After landing in Toronto, my father drove me straight to the hospital, much to Stella's relief, where they infused me with yet another dose of steroids in an attempt to reverse my rapidly declining platelet count. Dad sat next to my bed shaking his head and telling me off.

'You know, the Maple Leafs were versing the Montréal Canadiens tonight. Forty years since your birth and you're still causing me to miss important hockey games. I seriously worry that one of these days you're going to wake up dead.'

'Yes, Dad, but not today.'

'What I can't understand,' he said, rubbing his forehead in frustration, 'is why you took that drug when you knew there were so many risks.'

Ever the banker, my father was risk averse and had a difficult time understanding my seemingly reckless decisions.

'Dad, most people won't do Lemtrada because of the risks, but it's the only medically recognised drug at the moment that potentially offers a cure. With big risks come big rewards. Besides, as long as I do the mandated monthly blood tests, the side effects are manageable. Unlike MS, most of Lemtrada's side effects can be treated. I just screwed up and let them go too long. I blame it on the cabbage.'

Dad looked perplexed, then shrugged his shoulders and sighed.

'Kat, you've always fought hard for what you've believed in, even when you left home at 16. Whether you know it or not, I'm proud of you for giving this a shot. But please, just don't kill yourself in the process.'

Dad ruffled my hair and playfully punched me in the shoulder. Instantly, another bruise started to appear.

'Oh geez, sorry!'

As usual, there were no tears or hugs, emotions being a sign of weakness in our family, stiff British upper lip and all, but truth be told, I think we were both a little teary and emotional on the inside.

Stella and I returned to Australia a month after Christmas, and while my thyroid condition stabilised, my blood platelet count continued to be an ongoing concern. The steroids I was given should've knocked the ITP on its head, but they didn't. Weirdly, I felt fine—the only clue to my deteriorating condition was that I continued to look like I'd gone 12 rounds with Mike Tyson. I had huge, nasty-looking bruises all over my body.

I decided to go ahead with my plans to visit my friends Michael and Victoria in Melbourne for the weekend despite my scary appearance. The first night of my arrival, we settled in for pizza and a binge session of the TV series, *Ozark*. Around 10 p.m., my mobile unexpectedly rang. I hesitated before answering, knowing that late-night calls usually involved one of two things: bad news or sex. The latter was wishful thinking, even though I had now been divorced and single for more than five years.

'Is this Kat Finnerty?'

'Yes,' I replied as I held a tissue over my nose to catch the steadily dripping blood and put the call on speaker so I could hear it better.

'It's Gary from the Dorevitch lab. I'm sorry to call so late, but you need to know your lab results.'

'So to clarify, this is a blood call, not a booty call, right?'

'Excuse me?'

'Sorry, never mind. What are my lab results?'

'Well, your blood platelet count is one.'

I knew this wasn't good.

'Normal range is between 150 and 400, which means you're at severe risk of uncontrollable internal bleeding. Do you understand what I'm telling you? It doesn't get much worse than this. You need to seek medical attention immediately.'

'Gotcha.'

I thanked him and hung up. My friends stared at me with concern, having paused the final episode we were engrossed in.

I pointed to the remote.

'Can you please press play so I can at least see how this episode ends before I die.'

Silence. They were now shaking their heads in bewilderment. 'What?'

Okay, so I had to admit I was looking a little worse for wear. In addition to my massive bruises, my gums and nose were now seeping blood. But the upside was that I felt perfectly fine.

'I think we should take you to emergency,' Victoria announced in a concerned voice.

'I've got my haematologist's after-hours number. I'll give him a call,' I replied.

He wasn't available, but another specialist was. He agreed to send through a prescription of a high-dose corticosteroid, a drug designed to stop my immune system from killing me.

'Where are you?'

'I'm in East Melbourne.'

'I'll fax the script over now. Go to the pharmacy first thing in the morning. You are aware it's imperative you do this first thing, right?'

'Yes, thanks.'

I was hoping the pharmacy opened early so I could still make my 9 a.m. yoga class. To say I had a fatalistic view of life and death would be an understatement.

'See? All good,' I told my friends, explaining the specialist's advice. I smiled, exposing my blood-soaked gums, and began cleaning up the blood that had dripped onto the floor from my nose during the call.

'Now, let's find out how Jason Bateman launders all that Mexican drug money!'

Thanks to my Kat lives, I survived the night. The next morning, as promised, I went to the pharmacy and collected my prescription. Then it was on to my yoga class. I resigned myself to the moment. What will be, will be, I told myself. Sensibly, I gave the headstands a miss.

Let me explain my head space. In my world, doing yoga was a calculated risk, part of my holistic healing process to keep the mind and body strong. I wasn't reckless or suicidal, but I didn't wrap myself in cotton wool either. After years of living on the edge, I'd decided long ago not to let the fear of death stop me from doing the things I wanted to do. I did not want to die, but my biggest fear centred around not fully living. Thanks to my army days and the inspirational stories of my Czech Nana surviving WWII, I was a great believer in the 'what doesn't kill you makes you stronger' theory of life.

My haematologist called me into his office first thing Monday.

'I just saw your blood results and notes from the weekend. Sorry I wasn't on call. The haematologist you spoke to specialises in paediatrics. Kids can survive low platelet counts like yours, but not usually adults. How you didn't suffer a severe intestinal or brain haemorrhage is beyond me. You just dodged a bullet.'

Ah, Russian roulette, I knew this game! I was an expert at dodging bullets. I'd spent half my life pulling the trigger on various drug treatments and other alternative therapies, hoping it would cure rather than kill me.

The haematologist added, 'I've ordered you an infusion of intravenous immunoglobulin, better known as IVIG, from the blood bank. A courier will have it here shortly. My assistant has already booked you into the hospital next door.'

'Great, so crisis averted?' I asked hopefully.

'No, not even close. Kat, this is a very temporary measure. If the drug doesn't work, we're going to have to go down the path of surgery and operate.'

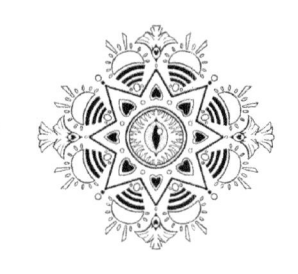

CHAPTER FORTY-FOUR
Zombie Apocalypse

My Zombie Apocalypse plan is simple but effective; I fully intend to die in the very first wave. Seems more logical than undergoing all kinds of hardships only to die eventually anyway, through bites, malnutrition or terminally chapped lips.
~ Graham Parke

I've always had a good relationship with my haematologist. He was a practical, no-nonsense kind of guy who told it like it was, no sugar-coating, and I liked that about him. But now he had me a little concerned because he was wearing his serious face.

'Okay...uh, hit me with it.'

'If we can't get on top of this platelet issue, we're going to have to do a splenectomy.'

'A what?'

'We're going to have to remove your spleen. It's a fist-sized organ that sits next to your stomach, up behind your left ribs. It removes and filters old and damaged blood cells and produces antibodies that help fight off infection. You can survive without one but it means you're more likely to develop dangerous infections later on in life like pneumonia and meningitis.'

He paused and gave me a chance to soak up the information. He was handing me yet another double-edged sword.

'Oh, and there can be complications from the operation itself—blood clot, hernia, inflammation of the pancreas, lung collapse—although the main issue is serious infection, which results in death in 50% of cases.'

His speech made me start comparing myself once again to the Black Knight. A knight who was now missing his thyroid, his spleen, his vision, the use of his arms and his legs, and who was slowly bleeding to death because he had no blood-clotting capability.

Black Knight: It's just a scratch, I've had worse!

King Arthur: Are you crazy?

Black Knight: Oh, I see. Running away, eh? Come back here and take what's coming to you! I'll bite your legs off!

King Arthur: Look, you stupid bastard, you've got no arms left!

Black Knight: Yes I have.

King Arthur: Look!

Black Knight: Just a flesh wound, a mere flesh wound.

Monty Python could have easily made a comedy sketch out of my life, it was so darkly humorous and ironic. I'd taken Lemtrada to stop losing the function of my body parts, and now I was losing body parts that weren't functioning properly.

I almost laughed at the sheer lunacy of it all. I forced my attention back to my doctor who was still talking.

'...however, given your other conditions I will put a request in to start you on a drug called Eltrombopag. It's subject to approval on a case-by-case basis because it's pricey—$3000 dollars per month—but it might just mean we won't have to remove your spleen. The downside is you may have to take the drug for the rest of your life.'

'And if I do nothing?'

'Then it's almost certain you will die. Kat, have you looked in the mirror lately?'

'Good point. Oh, just one other thing: Do you have any idea what the heck these are on my neck?' I gingerly removed a scarf. 'Yesterday these disgusting, painful blisters erupted.'

'That, I'm afraid, is shingles, a nasty side effect of having a lowered immune system. You really are in the wars, aren't you. I'll write you a prescription for Acyclovir.'

Ohh, the shingles were my fault. Back when I decided to take Lemtrada, they'd told me the shingles vaccine was part of the protocol. I'd baulked at it, mainly because I was already on so many drugs and I was convinced at the time they were simply ticking off boxes and over-prescribing out of excessive precaution. So I lied about having the injection. Now I was paying the karmic price.

As I relocated my car from the doctor's office to the hospital car park across the road, I caught a glimpse of myself in the rear-view mirror. I looked like an actor in a B-grade Zombie horror film. Massive angry blisters from the shingles were splashed across my neck, blood dripped from my nose and my body was covered in bruises. While having ITP caused me no physical pain, the shingles made up for this in spades. Bloody hell, they were freakin' painful!

'Kat,' I declared to my reflection, 'you are officially a disgusting mess!'

I was genuinely struggling to see the positive side of my situation. The simple fact was, I had to go on yet another powerful drug for my blood platelet issue, caused by taking the chemo drug Lemtrada to cure the MS, and now I was taking an antiviral drug to counteract the shingles caused by the steroids I'd taken to fix the ITP caused by the Lemtrada. It was a never-ending line of falling dominos, and I was always one domino too late to stop the chain reaction. Time to check myself into 'hotel hospital', as I liked to refer to it, and give myself a chance to reset through focused mediation, mindfulness and a powerful regime of modern drugs and medicine.

During the following weeks the doctors administered doses of intravenous immune globulin antibodies and started me on the Eltrombopag in a bid to stop my blood platelet count from plummeting. I was also given a dose of Acyclovir to clear up the shingles. I'd gone from the person who avoided drugs and needles at all costs to welcoming everything Big Pharma could throw at me in a bid to keep me alive and pain-free.

I studiously ignored the guillotine hanging over my spleen and concentrated on the things I had control over, like the thoughts in my head and the food in my body. *This too shall pass*, I lovingly reminded myself. I began some of my killer meditation and mindfulness moves, like conceptualising the feelings I experienced during the good times, when I felt like I could take on the world and everything was going right, and applying them to my present crisis. In essence, emotional scaffolding.

I imagined I was Daniel LaRusso in *The Karate Kid* being guided by a spiritual Mr. Miyagi. Wax on, wax off! I drank celery juice by the gallon and tackled my daily dilemmas and challenges using a series of mental katas. I used wisdom, discipline and courage to overcome fear, anger and ignorance and used flexibility and adaptability to transcend rigidity and conformity. I found these better deflected the blows aimed at my body and mind. I let go of unhealthy attachments and embraced the concept of impermanence with grace and understanding, knowing that while illness and death in life are inevitable, endless suffering is a choice. Hah! Ninja skills for showtime. As I collected my coloured belts of knowledge, I knew that if I had to face the final battle, the ultimate in showtime—death—then I'd be ready for it, a certified black belt in the most disastrous of disaster management.

Luckily it never came down to that. By the end of the fourth week, the drugs and my all-in approach worked their magic and I began to recover. The universe, karma, destiny, whatever you want to call it, in conjunction with several multinational pharmaceutical conglomerates, had once again seen fit to throw me a lifeline. It was a powerful reminder to be grateful for the country I lived in, a place where the healthcare system was advanced and generous enough to save me.

The only challenge I had now was being tethered to an incredibly expensive drug for the rest of my life. If there was one lesson I'd learnt about magic pills, it was that they always came with a price. It also meant I couldn't travel overseas for any extended period because the drug was only subsidised within Australia and required a quarterly sign-off.

Six months went by. I still felt good, so I made the decision to wean myself off the Eltrombopag. My haematologist Dr Rob was supportive but not optimistic about the plan working.

'That's not how the drug works, Kat, but you never know.'

I didn't let the odds stop me and once again went into dieting overdrive. I guzzled green juice and avoided refined, processed foods and sugars while keeping up a daily regime of yoga, meditation and exercise. Lo and behold, my platelet count didn't fall off a cliff but instead happily continued to thrive without the drugs coursing through my system. I was cured! Best of all, my MS had once again gone into remission. I'd finally managed to remove the right domino.

Looking back, as odd and twisted as the whole saga was, I never once feared dying. I just accepted if I died, I died and if I survived then it meant God, the Universe, Karma had other plans for me. Now it was time to figure out just what those plans were.

CHAPTER FORTY-FIVE
Bake a Cake for Someone You Hate

Be the person who breaks the cycle.
If you were judged, choose understanding.
If you were rejected, choose acceptance.
If you were shamed, choose compassion.
Be the person you needed when you were hurting,
not the person who hurt you.
Vow to be better than what broke you
To heal instead of becoming bitter
so you can act from your heart, not from your pain.
~ Lori Deschene

I slid the decadent mud cake out of the oven. An invisible cloud of chocolatey, sugary goodness filled the kitchen and wafted through the rest of my house. I'd baked the cake to celebrate the arrival of Trev and Tahlia's second baby, another girl. Four years had now passed since Trev walked out on me. My health issues were under control and I'd been in remission for six months since ditching the Eltrombopag. Although I had well and truly come to terms with Trev's new relationship, I was still struggling to accept the fact my ex-husband had chosen to start a whole new family. Especially when he already had three kids of his own!

Granted, he'd shacked up with a younger woman whose biological clock was ticking, but surely he realised that with two more kids, he would now have less time, attention and money to spend with our children. Turns out, they weren't interested in my opinion. Hence the cake.

Baking a cake is an act of kindness and love. It's a reward, a symbol of celebration and happiness. I could have sent them a card or put up a congratulatory Facebook post or completely ignored the event, but it wouldn't have been the same. A cake takes time and effort to make. It's personal, plus the mere act of baking the cake meant I could reflect on why I was doing it, in my case, planting karmic seeds of sweetness for my future rather than bitterness.

I did my best to mindfully imbue the batter with forgiveness and fold plenty of love and happiness into the frosting. I did not, as some friends jokingly suggested, lace it with poison. It's hard to share a cake and enjoy it with your ex-husband and his new partner if you all die a painful death. I even went so far as to try to kick off a new movement on Facebook and Instagram called #BakeaCakeforSomeoneYouHate. But the concept never took off. It seemed people didn't like baking cakes for people they hate. Pity.

Never Let a Good Disaster go to Waste

I called out to Stella to be ready in five minutes. My daughter, now 15, was attending the local high school—her choice, not mine—and that meant Trev was happy as well. She was a diligent student, and I absolutely loved having her home with me in Jrudgerie. The two older boys were still attending the nearby Catholic boarding school but came home every weekend. Trev and I had settled into an easy rhythm of sharing the care of the kids, although it had taken some time to work out. I had to swallow my pride and ease up on my rigid self-righteousness.

Many people assumed I'd be out of Jrudgerie the second Trev ditched me, but I wasn't about to leave my children behind or take them away from their father. I committed to staying in town until the kids finished school. Unlike Trev, I was still single and free as a bird. My divorce afforded me the freedom to pursue other passions, like yoga, spending time with my family in Canada and setting up new businesses. As I placed the cake into a box ready for transport, the intense smell of chocolate took me back to my first Easter after the breakdown of my marriage.

This was not an easy time in my life for me. I was suffering from a bout of debilitating loneliness that I couldn't seem to shake. Normally, I would have been with Trev, the kids and their cousins camping down at the beautiful Mornington Peninsula south of Melbourne. But of course I hadn't been invited that Easter. Tahlia had taken my place and was no doubt hiding Easter eggs, nibbling kabana and cheese by the fire, sipping on champagne, and cuddling up to Trev because it was always bloody freezing there this time of year.

Instead, I found myself home alone in Jrudgerie, stuffing my face full of sugar and sherry and feeling incredibly sorry for myself. My phone had not rung in days. To add insult to injury, I was torturing myself by scrolling through endless Facebook posts of happy families with chocolate egg collections so big parents would be dealing with hyper kids bursting with an excess of pimples for the next month. I knew I should've forced myself outside to do something—anything—but the weather was crap and the little devil on my shoulder convinced me to hibernate and self-medicate with cheap wine and half-eaten bunnies left behind by my kids.

Ethel, my sweet 80-year-old neighbour, was the only person to call round for a chat during this time, offering fresh scones and an invite to pop over to see her latest creation, a stuffed teddy bear she was making to raffle off at the hospital bazaar. But I blew her off, claiming I was busy with other chores. Chocolate and Easter it seemed, were quickly becoming synonymous with alcohol and bad decisions.

To be honest, I'd been managing okay up until this point, but the sudden onset and ferocity of the sadness had taken me by surprise. I'd not just fallen off the wagon, I'd been run over by it! So this was the downside to the post-breakup period, when all the attention faded away and the friends and family who'd initially rallied around you went back to their daily lives and their own families, leaving you to finish picking up the pieces.

Never Let a Good Disaster go to Waste

I was marinating in my own misery. Finally something snapped in my head and I screamed, 'Enough! Stop eating!' I told myself, *Sure, you're sad and lonely, but what are you going to do to pull yourself out of this?* Then it hit me. Why not start a company organising holidays for single parents and teens struggling in my exact same situation! The holiday would have to be an affordable, cool adventure, a detox from technology, and feature a connection to nature. Most of all, it would need to showcase a different culture and allow parents and kids to give back and help others less fortunate than themselves.

Inspired and emboldened by sherry and sugar, I booked a ticket to Bali and left the very next day to turn my idea into a reality. And, as things have a habit of doing in my life when I put my mind to it, all the pieces fell into place. I connected with the right people and Empowered Experience was born. I returned home to Jrudgerie a week later and noticed Ethel's blinds were down in the middle of the day. I asked another neighbour if she was away. The neighbour replied that poor Ethel had been so lonely she'd stopped eating and had become malnourished. The family felt it was best to admit her to the hospital for treatment.

The news was a hard slap in the face, a wake-up call. I was shocked and angry with myself. There I'd been all Easter, sitting in my house feeling sorry for myself, feeding my face with bunny ears, while poor, sweet Ethel had been starving herself to death next door, desperately reaching out for my attention. And I'd ignored her! I'd gone to Bali to find a purpose and set up a business designed to make a difference to people when all along there was a person living right next to me who I could've helped. I'd just been too selfish, self-absorbed and 'busy' to notice. Lama Marut used to say that depression and loneliness are forms of selfishness turned inward, that all the love and happiness we receive in the world is created by giving love and happiness to others, and in my case he was spot on.

This incident helped cement my resolve. I knew in order to be truly happy, I had to practise self-help through selflessness and think more about others. After visiting Ethel in hospital, I committed to dropping in on her more often and made it my mission to give back and do volunteer work with each group I took to Bali for Empowered Experience. I embraced Pablo Picasso's famous motto: 'The meaning of life is to find your gift. The purpose of your life is to give it away.'

And now here I was, three and half years after the Ethel incident, baking chocolate cakes for the lover of my ex-husband and booking my fifth retreat to Bali. Ash, the big-hearted southerner with the Matthew McConaughey good looks, would have been proud of me. The only issue still weighing heavily on me was that I wasn't even close to finishing my book, How to get Over Betrayal in 12 Hours. Despite the fact I'd been announcing to everyone that my goal was to complete it in the months following the end of my marriage. The truth was, I was failing terribly at the endeavour. It was incredibly frustrating. I wasn't one to make empty promises, well, not unless you count all the times I swore I'd never drink again. Maybe the answer was to make a dedicated trip to Ubud in Bali to find some inspiration.

After all, when you're a world-class procrastinator like me, only a journey to the island's spiritual and artistic heartland, the place where Elizabeth Gilbert wrote her book *Eat, Pray, Love*, would be enough to unleash the literary juices fermenting inside me.

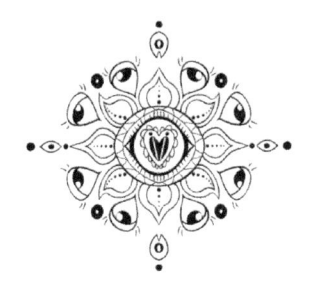

CHAPTER FORTY-SIX
A Shamanic Brush with Elizabeth Gilbert

Shamanic training involves a big spiritual cleanse. It is about strongly stepping into the path of love and trust, leaving behind energetic imprints and attachments we have outgrown that are more fear-based. It is a sacred and powerful journey of healing and awakening.
~ Mark Steinward, One Tribe Healing

It was late afternoon when my motorbike taxi pulled up to Jiwa's House, a classically designed Balinese homestay on the outskirts of central Ubud. It was located on a quiet, tree-lined street close to Radiantly Alive, the yoga studio where I liked to practise. All the rooms overlooked a lush tropical garden of fragrant frangipani and colourful bougainvillea interspersed with tiled fountains, carved stone statues and winding stone walkways.

Ubud itself was a larger reflection of the homestay, a stunningly beautiful town located about an hour's drive north of Denpasar, high on a mountain plateau. Everything about it was picture-postcard Bali, from the emerald-green rice terraces and steep, rainforest-covered ravines to the streets lined with ancient stone temples and a sacred forest full of cheeky monkeys. More importantly, Ubud was bursting with great food and kick-ass yoga teachers. It was my happy place and I hoped it would also soon be my writing salvation.

As evening approached, I strolled up a narrow pathway cut between rice paddies to one of my all-time favourite spots, Café Pomegranate. It overlooked a patchwork of immaculate green rice paddies that glistened in the setting sun. I ordered chicken satay on lemongrass sticks and a Bintang beer just as the sun was setting. The air was hot and humid, but I felt light, motivated and happy. I was committed to getting my book done.

It had been six years since I first started writing *'How to Get Over Betrayal in 12 Hours'* and I'd finally stashed enough cash to fund a dedicated trip to Bali just to complete the book. In the interim, I'd discovered some profound truths about myself.

Firstly, that true inner peace only visited me when I let go of my selfish desires and instead cultivated love, kindness and compassion for those around me. Fridge magnet cliché, I know, but I swear to God it's true! Secondly, that my happiness was highly dependent on how grateful and content I was in the here and now, not some imagined future or remembered past.

And thirdly, I could only maintain a positive outlook on life when I actively looked for the silver lining in every dark cloud and accepted that everything was perfectly imperfect, including me.

Michael J. Fox summed it up best when he said, 'If you don't think you have anything to be grateful for…take it from me, keep looking. Because you don't just receive optimism, you can't wait for things to be great and then be grateful for that. You've got to be behave in a way that promotes it.'

As I picked up my Bintang from the table and took a swig, mulling over my thoughts, I noticed two men sitting nearby. They smiled, held up their own Bintangs in a toast and beckoned me to come over and sit with them.

After introducing themselves as Mark and Dave from Perth, I quickly discovered one of them was hiding a fascinating secret behind his rugged, farm-boy good looks. Mark, it turned out, was an accredited shaman in the American-Indian tradition and ran retreats in Perth under the umbrella of his spiritual collective, 'One Tribe'. Mark didn't look remotely like a shaman, not that I was entirely sure what an American-Indian-Aussie shaman should look like. My imagination threw up images of a wild-eyed indigene with tribal tattoos and long hair. Mark had none of these attributes, but he did exude a gentle, intuitive wisdom. He explained to me that shamanism, in its purest form, created a bridge between the physical world and the spiritual dimension for healing, divination and transformation and that a lot of his work involved counselling people who suffered from emotional blockages and trauma in their lives.

'Kat, I met my first shamanic teacher in my early 20's and since then I've been on a long journey to heal myself and others.

And one of the most important things I've found is that our essence is pure and that healing is about releasing what is not us. We are not broken; we are whole and we can create a dream life for ourselves. I'm living proof of that.'

Hmmm, so if you were ever going on holiday in Bali and wanted to bask in the cliché of meeting a man claiming to be a conduit to the infinite knowledge and wisdom of the spirit world, Ubud was the place. I couldn't help but ask him what he thought of my quest to write a book designed to help people overcome suffering and betrayal in 12 hours. I added, for good measure, that I too was suffering a blockage, mostly of the literary rather than the emotional or intestinal variety.

He generously shared something profound with me—chalk one up for the shaman—about how he'd met Elizabeth Gilbert at an ashram in India while she was writing her memoir, *Eat, Pray, Love*. My jaw dropped open and I stared at him in wonder. Elizabeth Gilbert? What were the odds of running into a shaman who'd met the author of the book that had spurred me to come here in the first place? Mark revealed that in his chats with Liz, he'd learned she had also struggled with writer's block and putting pen to paper.

'Listen Kat, shamanic healing is very results focused. When you have an issue, we try resolving it on the table within that session, or perhaps at the most in a few follow-up sessions if we have to work through some deeper layers. You have to remember, everything is just energy—it can be moved, shifted, transformed. Which means every problem has a root energetic cause. If I were you, I'd try listening to your spirit guides more, their wisdom is immeasurable. And besides, if it only took you 12 hours to get over your husband's betrayal, then it should only take you 12 hours to write your frickin' book!'

Mark's blunt insight made me realise I needed to think about the root cause of my blockage and then sit my ass down, discover my flow and find 12 uninterrupted hours to write. Easy! For the next few days I tried to do just that. I just didn't count on Prue, my next-door neighbour—she could literally talk the leg off a chair—or the fact I was distracted by pretty much everything in Ubud: yoga, sound healings, raw food classes, movies, bike rides. My writing stalled despite Mark's inspirational pep talk. I was disappointed in myself. Surely there had to be a reason the universe led me here.

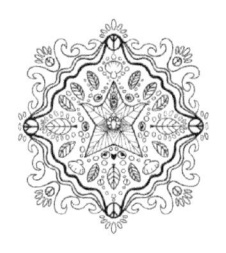

CHAPTER FORTY-SEVEN
Serendipity and Chocolate Cake

Ego says, 'Once everything falls into place, I'll feel peace.'
Spirit says, 'Find your peace and then everything will fall into place.'
~ Marianne Williamson

To say I was slightly preoccupied as I strolled to the yoga studio the next morning would be an understatement. My vision was filled with the myriad sights, sounds and smells of Ubud, and my mind was swirling with thoughts of my book and what Mark the Shaman had told me a few days earlier. As I stepped off the curb to cross the road, I felt a strong hand grab my arm and yank me backwards. A motorbike veered past, beeping wildly, its pillion passenger yelling angrily in Balinese. I gasped. Not because I'd just barely missed being hit by a motorbike for the second time in Bali but because my rescuer was the epitome of a tall, dark, handsome stranger. He was well over six and a half feet tall and had the clean-cut good looks, sparkling blue eyes and toned physique of an Olympic athlete.

'Oh,' I said, still in shock from both the near miss and his dazzling smile. 'You saved me from another hole in my leg.'

He stared at me, one eyebrow raised in confusion. Damn he was cute. He introduced himself as Alex and offered to walk me safely to the yoga studio. While we walked he asked what I was doing in Bali, other than dodging motorbikes. I laughed and filled him in on my intention to finish writing my book.

'Hmmm, I'm intrigued,' he replied, admitting he'd actually done a bit of writing himself. 'How about we catch up for dinner and you can tell me a little bit more about your project?'

I immediately agreed. *How good is this*, I thought. *A hero, a hunk and a writer? Kat, you are on a roll.*

The meeting proved to be as serendipitous as the encounter with Mark the Shaman. We connected over tempeh and tea where he offered to help put me on track with my book.

'That's so kind of you, Alex,' I replied gratefully, 'but, uh, I have a small problem. Ubud has too much going on. I'm way too distracted here. I need to go somewhere quieter and more secluded. I was thinking of a small island called Nusa Lembongan, southeast of Sanur.'

To my utter astonishment, he agreed to meet me there in a few days. I Googled him that night and discovered that not only had he published a number of business coaching books but had also written numerous articles for *Forbes* and *Fortune* magazine. He'd recently sold his start-up company in the US for seven figures. Wow, thank you Universe!

Never Let a Good Disaster go to Waste

My feet sank into the soft, white sand as I strolled to my favourite seaside café, Ginger and Jamu, overlooking picturesque Jungutbatu Beach on the island of Nusa Lembongan. The distinctive outline of Mount Agung volcano on Bali shimmered in the sea mist 50 km away. I ordered a chocolate cake and flipped open my laptop. Azure waves gently lapped at the shore, and a warm breeze rustled the fronds of the swaying palms above me.

I began working on a chapter of my book. Just behind the breaking waves a surfer waved at me and began paddling in on his shortboard. It was Alex. He'd been true to his word and had met me at the island a few days ago to help me with my writing. In the interim, I'd done a little more digging and found out he was a highly sought-after business coach who motivated and inspired people to achieve their best in life. I smiled and waved back. Life was good, actually better than good.

The cake arrived still steaming hot from the oven. I gratefully accepted it saying, 'Suksma,' to the petite Balinese girl, who in turn replied, 'Sama, sama,' her head bowed and her hands pressed together symbolically in front of her heart. I loved the Balinese culture; it was so beautiful. I lifted a teaspoon of the cake to my mouth and closed my eyes to savour the warm bittersweet flavour of chocolate mixed with coffee and ground almonds. Yum! The fact it was complemented by the coolness of a scoop of homemade vanilla bean ice cream elevated it into heavenly territory. What was it about me and chocolate in my life? It always seemed to mark important milestones and memories.

I glanced up and noticed Alex had made it to the beach and was chatting with Leona. She was a gorgeous, fit Aussie lady in her sixties who Alex and I had met a few days earlier. She happened to be staying in the same homestay as us, which consisted of three huts and a family-run warung. She had wavy blonde hair and blue eyes and reminded me of an older version of Bo Derek, minus the beaded braids. Although Leona was officially retired, she kept herself busy doing occasional gigs as a nude model for artists, a part-time actor, an aerobics instructor, and a copy editor. When she found out I was writing a book on overcoming the pain of betrayal, she offered to help. It was yet another miraculous coincidence and a sign I was on the right path.

I reined in my eternally wandering mind and refocused on the chapter I was currently working on, which I'd titled 'Gratitude'. I began typing: *My Buddhist teacher used to say, kindness teaches gratitude and, in turn, gratitude inspires kindness. Only if you've been kind to another person can you accept the idea that others can be kind to you. Gratitude is more than just appreciation, it's more than just sitting around saying thank you when someone does you a favour. It's about recognising all the good things happening in your life on a daily basis and creating the conditions that will lead to these outcomes. If you're grateful every day, if you're planting the right karmic seeds, it's hard to stay depressed and lonely.*

I took another bite of the chocolate mocha cake, satisfied with my writing effort so far. Alex sank down into the bamboo chair next to me, his perfectly cropped brown hair still wet from his recent surf on nearby Shipwrecks surf break. He was wearing a sleeveless top that showed off his impressively toned physique. I held out my fork containing a large piece of cake.

'Chocolate?' I offered with a cheeky grin, waving it back and forth in front of his face. He smiled back at me, the tiny lines around the edges of his clear blue eyes crinkling with amusement.

'How can I resist,' he laughed, and devoured the cake. 'So where are you up to today?'

I filled him in on the chapter. 'Do you know what the secret is to being happy and having it all?' I asked.

'Enlighten me,' Alex responded, leaning back in his chair.

'Knowing that you already do.'

He grinned and replied, 'Kat, I knew there was a reason why I rescued you from certain death. Maybe I need your words just as much as you need mine.'

For the next week Alex did his best to provide me with a framework and structure for my book, while Leona worked on crafting my writing style, punctuation and literary skills. Alex proved to be smart, attentive and understanding. He had the uncanny ability to ask the right questions and then counter all my problems with perfectly tailored solutions.

Although he didn't freely reveal much about himself, he admitted he'd had a recent experience that made him rethink everything in his life. He still loved his wife and was committed to her, but they'd agreed to have some time apart while he set off on a quest to find a deeper sense of peace, meaning and purpose. Oh well, there goes my tropical island romance, I thought. Why, oh, why do I put my trust in psychics? Unless, of course, by some miracle there happened to another tall, dark, handsome "Alex" on another tropical island somewhere. I laughed at the absurdity of the thought.

Conversely, Leona and I instantly recognised each other as kindred spirits and became good friends. She was like me in so many ways. She loved yoga, health and nutrition, she was divorced with one son, she was spiritual and adventurous, and she was also the number one pick for men in her age group on Tinder. Okay, so I wasn't close to being a top pick on Tinder, but the rest was on point.

With Leona and Alex by my side, I made serious headway, though I now realised the book was definitely not going to be a 12-hour affair. After a week of working, riding around the island on scooters and drinking sunset cocktails at The Deck restaurant, it was time to go our separate ways. Alex was meeting his wife in Europe, Leona had a dog-sitting gig in the Noosa hinterland and I needed to go home to my kids. It was an emotional goodbye as we stood on the beach under the fiery sun awaiting the ferry back to Bali. Alex smiled down at me, one of his massive hands resting on my shoulder.

'You've got this Kat, you just gotta rein that bitch in and stay focused.'

Leona gave me a big hug and a stern pep talk. 'Go home and finish the book. Then come to Queensland and I'll edit it for you. I've got a little window of time I can put aside for you while I'm dog-sitting. You can stay with me, which means you have three weeks to get your book together.'

'You can do it Kat,' chimed in Alex, 'You have more stories than the Empire State Building.'

We all cracked up laughing and hugged as salty tears and sweat streamed down our faces.

'I promise, I'll be there Leona, one way or another I'll make sure this book is in the bag!'

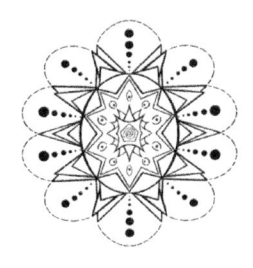

CHAPTER FORTY-EIGHT
It Starts with a Belief

Your beliefs become your thoughts
Your thoughts become your words
Your words become your actions
Your actions become your habits
Your habits become your values
Your values become your destiny
~ Mahatma Gandhi

I flew back to Melbourne from Bali, cradling my laptop with my unfinished manuscript in my arms and lugging a suitcase full of memories. The words of Leona, Alex and Mark the Shaman were still fresh in my mind, along with the images and tastes of Ubud and Nusa Lembongan.

I now had a mission and a timeline to work to—three weeks to finish the manuscript of *How to Get Over Betrayal in 12 Hours* and get my butt up to the Sunshine Coast in Queensland for the edit. So far it had only taken me six years, *pfssst*, what was another three weeks!

The following days were a blur as I worked on my manuscript and spent time with my kids. The new school year was fast approaching, and I scrambled to organise uniforms, shoes, socks, and jocks. I thought about how fortunate I was to have cultivated a good relationship with Trev and Tahlia since the divorce. The fact Trev was happy in Jrudgerie and that his partner was willing to embrace my kids in their home gave me the freedom to come and go at will. I wondered if I would have been as understanding had the roles been reversed. I explained to my kids that I needed to go to Queensland for a while to catch up with my editor and put the finishing touches on my book. Being teenagers, Jack, Luke and Stella didn't need me nearly as much as my ego wanted them to. They'd been brought up from an early age to be resilient, capable and self-sufficient and were used to me shooting off around the world. They knew I loved them to bits and that I would always be there for them—they only had to ask. I also wanted to impart on them the importance of doing whatever it takes to fulfil your life's passion.

'So if your book is a best-seller, does that mean we all get a big inheritance and you'll stop buying us second-hand jocks?' asked Jack.

Kids, they wield the truth like a samurai sword.

I arrived on the Sunshine Coast to beautiful warm weather and a clear blue sky. Leona greeted me with a hug, her latest

Never Let a Good Disaster go to Waste

Tinder date in tow. Her dog-sitting gig was located a little way outside of Noosa, in the rolling green hills of Cooran. A perfect distraction-free spot to complete my writing. However, Leona, being so much like me, wasn't a fan of sitting and working on a book for long periods of time. In between bouts of intense writing and editing, we did yoga, swam and body-surfed the waves at the beach, hiked to the rugged cliffs of Hell's Gate in Noosa National Park, and went on Harley rides to Maleny and Eumundi and other nearby small towns with her bikie friends.

While stopping for lunch at the Rainbow Beach pub on one of these rides, I realised I was looking across at Fraser Island, where 22 years earlier my trio of Irish men had gone four-wheel driving while I stayed behind trying to heal the hole in my leg. I reached down and rubbed the scar where the hole used to be. Although it and my soul had long since healed, I still had a nice round indentation as a reminder of those wonderful but challenging times. Leona, noticing me lost in thought, asked if I was okay. I told her the whole story of my Bali motorbike accident, my adventures with the Irish lads and my doomed relationship with a Scottish doctor and how this had irrevocably led me to Trevor.

'So do you believe in karma, fate or destiny?' she asked.

I sat back and thought about it carefully. 'I believe that every day, in every moment, I have the power to change my future.'

'In what way?'

'Well, I can choose to be compassionate and thoughtful when responding to adverse situations or I can overreact and let my emotions take control. I can choose to blame the world around me for my problems or I can accept personal responsibility for how my life is playing out and do something about it. Karma gives me a certain amount of control to shape my future, because everything is cause and effect, so what I choose to put out into the universe should theoretically be returned to me. And I'm proof that no matter how many times you screw up, no matter how many obstacles are placed in your path, it's never too late to change the pathway forward.'

'Amen sister, I'll drink to that! Here's to being in charge of our own destiny instead of being a victim of it.'

A few days later, while having a coffee at one of the trendy cafés lining Hastings Street in Noosa, destiny or karma chose once again to step into my life, this time in the form of a striking lime-green Saab convertible driving past.

'That looks just like my friend Klaas's car,' exclaimed Leona.

Leona strained her neck trying to get a better view of the driver. 'He has a house here in Noosa, but most of the time he lives on a tropical island in Vanuatu, somewhere out there in the South Pacific. I wonder if he's back.'

Vanuatu? Where the hell was Vanuatu? Moments later Leona's mobile rang. It was Klaas. In what turned out to be a case of pure coincidence he'd chosen that exact moment to ring Leona, unaware of his proximity to her. He explained he'd just returned to Oz and was booked in for a colonoscopy the next day. Could she possibly pick him up from the hospital as his partner was still in Vanuatu? Leona warmly agreed to help, and I volunteered to go along.

We pulled up at the private hospital the following day, and an older man in his sixties with a full head of greying hair, a prominent nose and wire-framed glasses gingerly sank into the front seat.

After giving Leona a big hug, he turned to me. 'And who the hell are you, young lady?'

'I'm Kat. I usually teach yoga, fitness and nutrition, but I'm taking time off to write a book called *How to Get Over Betrayal in 12 Hours.*'

'Is that so,' Klaas responded, bemused.

'Yes, I thought I'd be able to wrap it up in a bit over 12 hours, but I'm easily distracted, which may explain why after six years I haven't finished.'

He looked at me incredulously. 'You're kidding, right?'

'No, it's possible to get over betrayal in 12 hours if you have the right mindset.'

'No, I mean are you really using my colonoscopy appointment as an excuse not to work on your book today?'

I looked at him sheepishly. 'Ah, um, yep, I guess so.'

He laughed. 'You're a crack-up Kat! So do you have a publisher lined up for this book of yours yet?'

'I wish! I haven't thought that far ahead. I've been too—'

'Distracted? Yes, I'm starting to get the picture.'

'He turned to Leona. 'And you're copy editing this book for her?'

Leona nodded, her eyes sparkling with mischief.

'But you're just as easily distracted as she is!'

We looked at each other and laughed.

'Okay, listen, I have a great idea. My doctor just told me I need to lose some weight and get fit. I'm here for the next month or so. Why don't you help me shed some kilos and get in shape, and in return you can stay at my beach shack and I'll help with your book.' He paused. 'I used to dabble in publishing, you know. In fact, I published Hutton Gibson's book. You've probably heard of his son, Mel?'

'You mean Mel Gibson?'

'Yep.'

I looked at Leona and she shot me a reassuring wink.

'Deal!' I yelled, not realising this would turn out to be yet another sliding door moment in my life.

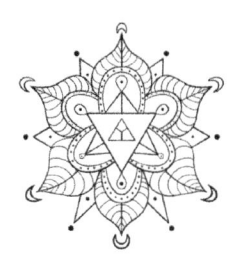

CHAPTER FORTY-NINE
Never Let a Good Disaster Go to Waste

Yesterday I was clever, so I wanted to change the world.
Today I am wise, so I am changing myself.
~ Rumi

Klaas lived at one of the most sought-after addresses in Noosa, a suburb called Sunshine Beach. The 'shack' was actually an architecturally designed two-storey residence perched on the edge of a cliff overlooking an endless stretch of pristine white sand beach. When he wasn't there he rented it out to rich executives and holidaying politicians. It was spectacular.

I took on the task of whipping Klaas into shape very seriously. I prepared all his meals and scheduled daily walks as well as regular body-weight training sessions and stretching. It wasn't too hard to find the inspiration to exercise and get outside.

Sunshine Beach stretched 20 km down the coast to Point Arkwright at Coolum Beach and north to the rocky promontories of Noosa National Park and the isolated cove of Alexander Bay. We exchanged stories as we walked, me stumbling sporadically as I shared with him the disasters and triumphs that had occurred in my life: my mum's death, overcoming MS, my discovery of Buddhism, yoga and meditation. Klaas reminded me of my dad in many ways. He had a confident, superior manner and very precise views on how the world should work.

One day after reading one of the 12 principles I had written, Klaas shook his head and announced, 'You know Kat, this is wrong, it's all wrong.'

'Which bit?' I asked, trying to think of the paragraph I needed to change.

'All of it! You need to stop writing a "how to" manual and instead tell the story of your life.'

'But...but that's not what this book is about. Besides, why would anyone want to read a story about my life?'

'You've talked my ear off these last few days. Just start at the beginning and go from there. You have an amazing and inspiring story to tell.'

That night I couldn't sleep. I agonised over the fact that not only would I have to start my book all over again, but I'd also have to share my innermost thoughts and demons with the world. I'd be opening myself up to judgement and criticism. Could I really do that? The answer was yes, if it meant people could relate to me and understand that even if you screw up, you can still find a way out of the cycle of suffering. Klaas was right. My story was never solely about the 12 steps or about the destination of 'getting over betrayal'. It was more about the journey and how we perceive our circumstances along the way. I knew if I was going to do this right, my book had to incorporate my whole journey, not just a small part of it. It had to be an honest portrayal of my far-from-perfect life, the mistakes I made, the lessons I learned, the spiritual and philosophical journey I embarked on to become happy and content.

Somewhere in the early hours of the morning I dozed off and woke up with the sun illuminating my room in a golden glow. For a minute I thought I was back in Jrudgerie all those many years ago when I'd watched the sunrise the morning after my betrayal. Then I heard Klaas calling out, ready for his early morning power walk, and reality came flooding back. I rang Leona and told her about my epiphany and my decision to start over. She wasn't thrilled but she understood.

'Kat, you know I love you and believe in what you're trying to achieve, which is why I was happy to help. But I can't edit a moving target. When you're done, bring me the finished copy and I'll look at it again.'

Klaas, on the other hand, was ecstatic. 'You've made the right decision, Kat. You know it in your heart.'

When we returned from our walk, he made coffee and handed me a plate with some Vegemite on toast. 'Breakfast?'

I cast my gaze skyward and chuckled as the words of Pema Chodren, one of my favourite Buddhist nuns, sprang to mind: 'Nothing ever goes away until it teaches you what you need to know.'

'What's so funny?'

'Karma, destiny, fate. Sometimes you spend your whole life hating something only to realise you could have chosen to love it instead.'

Klaas looked at me, mock horror in his eyes. 'How on earth could anyone possibly hate Vegemite?'

I shrugged, 'I guess it's just a matter of perception.'

Later that afternoon, as the sun was setting, I wandered out to the wooden table on the back deck and sat down to admire the endless expanse of blue ocean stretching to the horizon. I placed my laptop gently in front of me. In the distance, I spotted a sailboat tacking through the waves while a lone seagull wheeled elegantly in the breeze. I took a deep breath, opened the laptop and began typing out the story of my life. The words, for once, began to flow without effort.

I've come to the realisation that life is like a jigsaw puzzle. Some parts are simple, with obvious corners and straight sides; others have jagged edges and are difficult to figure out. It doesn't help to get angry at a puzzle piece when it doesn't fit, and you can't force it. Jigsaw puzzles don't necessarily come together in any specific order, but if you know in your heart of hearts that every piece has its rightful place and that its purpose will be revealed to you in time, then you can surrender to the process and cultivate patience and acceptance. Eventually, you realise that even the most difficult pieces, the ones punishingly hard to decipher and place, can actually provide you with immense satisfaction and joy and be the key to completing the overall picture. They help make the puzzle whole.

I paused and stopped typing. I had now reached a point in my life where I could accept each piece of my life's puzzle for what it was: a small, important part of a greater whole. I'd manage to overcome my betrayal in 12 hours not because I was somehow special or gifted but because I'd applied the life lessons and realisations I'd learned from the innumerable disasters of my past to transform the suffering and pain of my present. In essence, I'd never let a good disaster go to waste.

And with that, my new book was born.

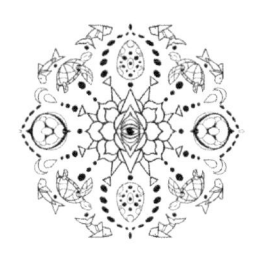

EPILOGUE
Tales of the South Pacific

I wish I could tell you about the South Pacific. The way it actually was. The endless ocean. The infinite specks of coral we called islands. Coconut palms nodding gracefully towards the ocean. Reefs upon which waves broke into spray, and inner lagoons, lovely beyond description. I wish I could tell you about the sweating jungle, the full moon rising behind the volcanoes, and the waiting. The waiting.
The timeless, repetitive waiting.
~ James A. Michener

'What is that?' I wondered aloud as I gazed out the plane's window. Shimmering in the endless deep blue of the Pacific Ocean was an impossibly long, turquoise-green ribbon, looking for all the world like an iridescent, watery mirage.

'It's a ribbon reef. Magical isn't it?' said a man's voice from the seat behind me. His accent was unusual, undeniably Australian, but with a slight American twang.

'Yes,' I replied, 'it's breathtakingly beautiful.'

The woman sitting next to me leaned over to look, and seeing the reef added, 'That's the far northern tip of New Caledonia's outer reef system. You're looking at the second largest barrier reef in the world, outside of the Great Barrier Reef, of course.'

I shook my head in bewilderment. The world was full of beauty and wonder, and some of its most precious jewels lay hidden in the vast blueness of the Pacific. Just like the place where I was heading now, the mystical islands of Vanuatu. All I knew about the island chain was what I'd just read in the in-flight magazine: that it was almost 1,200 km long, featured half a dozen active volcanoes, was once populated by cannibals, and was popular with cruise ships for its rich diverse culture and relatively untouched outer islands. Oh, and it was home to Klaas's cocoa, coffee and coconut plantation.

I returned to reading the article. It featured the Jordan River gorge on the island of Espiritu Santo, the largest island in Vanuatu. The photos were incredible: towering limestone walls, impossibly high waterfalls and fierce, colourful tribesmen wearing nothing but loincloths. It was remote, wild and pristine—the perfect adventure for my next retreat with Empowered Experience. I made a mental note to look up the author, Alex Bortoli, when I arrived in Santo.

Exactly how and why I found myself winging it to Vanuatu started two months earlier, when Klaas called me from his plantation on tiny Aore Island, just off Santo.

'Kat, she left me! My partner left me. I found out she's been planning it for months,' he lamented, clearly distraught.

'Well it's a damn good thing you've been helping me with a book about how to get over betrayal,' I replied, attempting to sound upbeat. 'You might want to reread a few chapters of my memoir.'

'Hmmm, good point.'

We chatted, and Klaas calmed down enough to ask me how it was going with the writing. I explained I still had a few chapters to go.

'It's like an unfinished painting, I'm always trying to add another brush stroke to make it perfect.' I sighed with exasperation. 'But I've made the decision not to do any more paid work until my book is finished.'

Klaas commented on the very real possibility of me living on baked beans for the rest of my life. I reminded him to never let a good disaster go to waste.

Two weeks later I called Klaas to see how he was doing. As it turned out, he was beyond okay—he was bordering on the euphoric.

'You're not going to believe it Kat', he exclaimed. 'I've met the most wonderful lady, Vinnie. She's a former Miss Vanuatu contestant. We're living together now.'

'Well, I'll be damned. Sounds like you certainly didn't waste any time letting your disaster go to waste. Well done!'

'You have to meet her! She's smart, funny and beautiful. You'll love her. In fact, why don't you come over for Christmas? We'll put the finishing touches on your book, and you can bring one of those fancy Thermomix cooking machines over to jazz up our menu. Maybe you can even make some chocolate from the plantation's cocoa trees!'

I gave his suggestion some serious thought, although my go-to response was 'Hell yeah!' In terms of my overall health, I was feeling 100% better compared to where I'd been a few years earlier. I was confident the chemo drug Lemtrada I'd taken five years previously had done its job and wiped out my rogue immune cells. With regard to the CCSVI Liberation Therapy, the results from the trial were inconclusive. I couldn't be sure whether it had helped me or not, but there was no denying my balance and gait had now improved to the point where I could confidently walk a decent distance without falling or tripping. Sure, I still had other minor issues: my thyroid sometimes played up, I had chronic pain in my lower back due to the deterioration of my spine and my left arm was still weaker than my right. But I didn't view any of these problems as problems. I thought of them as 'opportunities'. I felt like I was winning at the game of life.

As for my kids, I'd just agreed to let Trev have them for the second Christmas in a row as they'd all been invited to a huge family gathering in Lorne on the Great Ocean Road. I knew they wouldn't want to miss out on a beach holiday with their cousins, it would have been selfish of me to object. Of course, this meant I'd once again be alone for the holidays, and if I stayed in Jrudgerie I'd undoubtedly end up repeating my Easter debacle, except instead of bingeing on chocolate and sherry I'd pig out on eggnog and fruitcake. A trip to Vanuatu would fit in perfectly.

The fibreglass banana boat powered through the sparkling blue-green chop of the Segund Channel separating Aore Island from Espiritu Santo. I stood at the bow, my arms spread wide, and each time the salt spray cascaded over me I screamed with delight. Klaas laughed. He'd just picked me up from the airport half an hour earlier and knew I enjoyed a thrill, so he was gunning the boat through the swells on purpose.

'Welcome to Santo!' he yelled. 'An island populated by misfits, mercenaries and missionaries. The ultimate sunny place for shady characters!'

I laughed and ducked under the spray from a large wave. It was a divine tropical day, and the jungle-clad hills of Freshwater Plantation rose ahead of us. As we pulled up to the jetty, the water turned to aquamarine glass. I watched as a cloud of tropical reef fish scattered into the shadows of the pier. From underneath the shade of a nearby palm tree, a stunning Ni-Vanuatu lady strolled out to greet us. She had a vibrant red hibiscus in her hair and was wearing a colourful island dress.

'Kat, meet Vinnie. Vinnie, meet Kat."

I looked at Klaas and mouthed, 'She's gorgeous!'

He winked and smiled at me.

Vinnie kissed me on both cheeks and welcomed me by gently placing a pink hibiscus flower in my hair.

'Welcome to Freshwater, Kat. Welcome to paradise.'

Klaas grabbed my bag and ushered me forward. 'Come on Kat, let's get you settled in your room.'

My room turned out to be a beautiful traditional farè with a natangora palm-thatched roof and floor to ceiling glass bifold doors and windows facing the ocean. A small wooden balcony overlooked my own private beach. A bathroom connected to the side of the bungalow featured an open air shower. The view from the deck was stunning, all sparkling water overhung with native burao trees covered in pink and yellow flowers.

'After you've unpacked come up and join us at the house for a martini. Just follow the signs,' Klaas said, gesturing to the carved wooden Freshwater Plantation signs nailed to the trees outside.

I unpacked my bag, removed my iPad and walked onto the shaded balcony. I marvelled at the colourful vista that stretched out before me, a watercolour painting of different shades of blues and greens, as I sunk into a padded chair and began typing a blog:

So beautiful here ☺
I wonder what exciting adventures await me?
Will I live blissfully in paradise, or will I stumble into yet another disaster?
The point being, it doesn't really matter, does it?

My life's always been about the journey, not the destination. Who wants a fairy-tale ending anyway? Boring! Life should be an adventure, a roller coaster ride, a jigsaw puzzle. Some place where you never know your next destination or how you're going to get there or when the next piece of the puzzle will show up to complete the picture.

Whatever happens, I plan to enjoy every last minute of the ride.

As for my book, my goal is to finish it here in Vanuatu, once and for all. Sure, it may have started out as a simple 12-step self-help book, but thanks to Klaas, it's now morphed into my life story. I'm feeling comfortable about baring my soul and sharing all my 'aha!' moments. Why? Because it's never been about my pride or ego, or becoming famous, or turning myself into a preacher or guru or self-help prophet. Rather, it's because I know how much of a difference the concept of 'never letting a good disaster go to waste' has made in my own life and I want to share it with everyone. No one should have to suffer for a minute longer than they need to. Buddha once said,

> *In the end, these things matter most...*
> *How deeply did you love?*
> *How fully did you live?*
> *How well did you let go?*

And looking back over my life, I can say, with all honesty, I did love deeply, I did live fully, I did let go. My sincerest hope is that my thoughts, words and actions will resonate with someone out there and inspire them to throw off their own cloak of victimhood and claim back their freedom and peace in their heart. If I can even help to change one person's future for the better, then my mission will be complete.

Right now, in this moment...I am at peace. I am happy and content. Maybe it won't stay this way and that's okay too. I'm not perfect, but I can always strive to be better and my disasters help me to achieve this. Which is why I will continue to live by my rules. I'm certain they will keep me on the right path, a path full of laughter, love and the occasional scoop of chocolate ice cream! As Lama Marut would say, 'Om, I am enough. I have enough. A hum.'

Kat's Four Rules for Life

Always act from a place of love and kindness.
Always be aware of your perceptions.
Always embrace a radical acceptance of life.
AND
Never, never let a good disaster go to waste.

Love, Light and Kisses
KAT
Aore Island, Espiritu Santo, Vanuatu

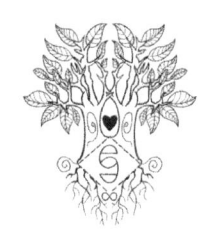

Want to find out what happens next in Vanuatu?

Head to my website www.katfinnerty.com for a sneak peek of my follow-up book, *Kat's Tales of the South Pacific: Life in the Most Disaster Prone Country on Earth*. It expands on my crazy disaster-prone life in Vanuatu (coping with earthquakes, tsunamis, cyclones and exploding volcanoes) and provides a tantalising glimpse into my blossoming tropical love story. Wohoo!

Printed in Great Britain
by Amazon